MARCO PREVIERO was born in Montpellier, France, in 1972. He moved to the UK in 1988 to finish his schooling – and stayed. Having long accepted without too much remorse the gentle pleasures of an uneventful and ordinary life, he was woefully unprepared to guide and support his seven-year-old daughter through the vicious agony of cancer treatment when she was diagnosed with a malignant brain tumour in April 2013. He has been trying his best to be a good father ever since.

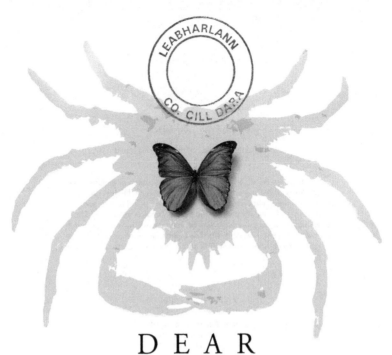

# DEAR
# MILLIE

DIARY OF A
SEVEN YEAR OLD
WITH CANCER

MARCO PREVIERO

Matador
9 Priory Business Park
Kibworth Beauchamp
Leicestershire LE8 0RX, UK
Tel: (+44) 116 279 2299
Fax: (+44) 116 279 2277
Email: books@troubador.co.uk
Web: www.troubador.co.uk/matador

ISBN 978-1784622-022

British Library Cataloguing in Publication Data.
A catalogue record for this book is available from the British Library.

Printed and bound in the UK by TJ International, Padstow, Cornwall
Typeset in Aldine by Troubador Publishing Ltd

**Matador** is an imprint of Troubador Publishing Ltd

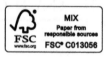

*To Millie, who has, despite her young age, guided me throughout this ordeal, and inspired me to keep going when hope was a currency I could not afford to use.*

*To Mr J – Millie's neurosurgeon – whose judgment, decision-making and skills were the single most instrumental and contributory factors in saving Millie's eyesight and, on the balance of probabilities, her life.*

*To the student nurses, nurses and senior nurses of Koala Ward (Great Ormond Street Hospital). In our darkest hours, you made all the difference.*

*Chapter headings are extracts from Henry F. Carey's translation of The Divine Comedy (Harvard Classics, Vol 20 – PF Collier & Son Company 1909–14).*

# CONTENTS

II – Purgatorio (*Purgatory*)

III – Paradiso (*Heaven*)

# INTRODUCTION

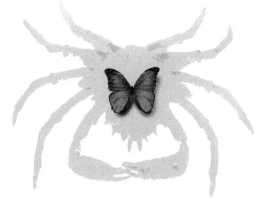

# Dear Millie,

I am writing you this letter in the hope that life has afforded you the opportunity to grow old enough to read it. Shortly after your seventh birthday you were diagnosed with a secreting germ cell tumour, a rare and malignant cancer of the brain, which initially manifested itself when you complained of 'fuzziness' in your beautiful brown eyes on the morning of 5th April 2013. The fuzziness, I quickly established, turned out to be loss of vision in your right eye and near-blindness in your left one.

Within the next two days you had undergone your first eight-hour craniotomy (brain operation) to preserve the little vision you had left. Within four days, by now blind, you were diagnosed with cancer, and within a fortnight you had begun your first cycle of aggressive chemotherapy. Over the course of the six months that followed, you would undertake two further brain operations, three additional cycles of chemotherapy and thirty sessions of radiotherapy 4,000 miles away from home.

The events that unfolded during that year were the most traumatic, upsetting and painful events in your life, in my life, in your mother's life and in pretty much all of our family's lives combined. To keep my sanity, I started writing what was happening to us as a family, and what was happening to you as my daughter. In doing so, I wanted to preserve the detail, so easily forgotten, of what you had to go through, and the courage with which you did it, so that you could read your story at an age when you would understand how extraordinary you had been during that time.

If you are reading this letter and diary now, then you have lived to tell the tale: a tale of courage, of fortitude, of resilience, of pain, of destruction, and, ultimately, of rebirth.

When hope was a currency I could not afford to use, in places sunlight could not reach, you rescued me out of the dark hell that is cancer when it creeps slowly, unstoppable, towards a loved one; and one so young. And so I felt it was fitting that I should use one of the most famous epic poems, *The Divine Comedy*, to help me narrate the events that unfolded during 2013, with you, rather than Virgil, as my guide.

**Hell** (Inferno) describes perhaps the most violent period of your illness: the discovery of the tumour and your first brain operation. Fear, uncertainty and shock were the dominant themes. Would you regain your eyesight? Would you live long enough for the medical profession to attempt to cure this most destructive of diseases? Would you remain the Millie May we had grown to love so much?

In **Purgatory** (Purgatorio) you will read how chemotherapy affected you, and why you had to undertake two further brain operations. We knew by now what we were facing. We knew it could eventually end your life. Much doubt remained: would your cancer be sensitive to the wave of cytotoxic drugs that were going to be systematically injected directly into your bloodstream over four months? How successful would the neurosurgeon be in removing the whole of the cancerous lump that was set deep within your brain? How would it affect some of the vital areas responsible for pumping out hormones essential for coping with day-to-day life?

And, finally, **Heaven** (Paradiso), which saw us move lock, stock and barrel 4,000 miles away from home, with your brother and sister in tow – so you could receive one of the most advanced radiotherapy treatments in the world over the course of nine weeks: proton beam. Treatment that would nonetheless cause some permanent damage to healthy brain matter and affect you cognitively; treatment that would alter your ability to produce your own growth hormones; treatment that could, in time, cause further malignancies in your brain…

What choice did we have? What alternative courses of action were available? Cancer kills and you had it. In attempting to cure it, we needed to provide the most beneficial treatment with the lowest risk. 'Most beneficial treatment' and 'risk' were both relative and contextual. There was no black and white in that game of life and death. We knew that in curing cancer we were going to cause irreparable damage that would alter your quality of life in a way we could not easily predict, and make you significantly worse before possibly making you better – because with the alternative there simply was no quality of life.

I hope we managed to weather the storm that descended with such brutal force into our lives, that 5th April 2013. I hope your mother and I were up to the task; we certainly tried our best. I hope you will look back at this period with a deep sense of pride and achievement in how you handled it all with the minimum of fuss. I hope you will realise how proud your mother and I are of you, then and now, and every minute in between. And, finally, I hope you will always remember the love of a father who never doubted his commitment to get you out of the grips of cancer and who will always carry your heart in his heart. This is your story.

*Daddy*

# I

## INFERNO
### (*HELL*)

"Nel mezzo del cammin di nostra vita
mi ritrovai per una selva oscura
ché la diritta via era smarrita."

*"When I had journeyed half of our life's way,
I found myself within a shadowed forest,
for I had lost the path that does not stray."*

Dante Alighieri, The Divine Comedy
*Inferno – Canto I, lines 1-3*

"Bad news, I'm afraid. It's a brain tumour."

Millie's paediatrician
*6) Day 1 – 12:35pm, Friday 5ᵗʰ April 2013*

# ALL HOPE ABANDON,
# YE WHO ENTER HERE

## 1) Day 1 – 7:12am, Friday 5ᵗʰ April 2013

Not quite the night before Good Friday, but close. This morning my seven-year-old daughter, Millie, woke up complaining of 'fuzziness' in her eyes. She had been feeling unwell for a couple of days, so, having just returned from our Easter break visiting my parents in Italy, we (we being my wife Vanessa and I) booked an appointment with our paediatrician up in London for later on today. By unwell, I don't mean anything spectacular. I mean the kind of 'unwell' that children all over the world, including my own three, experience from time to time, but generally sleep off. Still, call it luck, parental intuition, serendipity or coincidence, the appointment was booked for today to make sure nothing was brewing before the start of term.

Complaining of fuzziness in the eyes can be an indication of a variety of ailments. Certainly, come to think of it, Millie had suffered a particularly bad headache a month ago. It was something that went pretty much as quickly as it came, but maybe the two were related. Or maybe she needed glasses. I remember that we had thought about taking her to A&E (for the headaches, rather than possibly needing glasses), but decided against it on the basis that a little sleep had sorted the problem out. Vanessa was probably keener than me, but I reminded her that we took our eldest daughter, Ellie Rose, to A&E when she was four or five months old for what turned out to be nothing more than rhinopharyngitis (the common cold). Indeed, of the many child-related trips we made to our local A&E over the years, with the possible exception of an allergic reaction to pumpkin seeds (don't ask...) and eating a washing-up capsule full of detergent (helpfully made to look like something really yummy by a moronic dishwasher company), none turned out to be life threatening: far from it.

## 2) Day 1 – 7:15am, Friday 5th April 2013

So, back to the fuzziness. After a couple of relatively unscientific but nonetheless effective 'How many fingers am I holding up?' tests, it becomes apparent that Millie has lost vision completely in her right eye ("I can just see brown, Daddy") and has retained very limited vision in the left. I find it difficult to even write that last sentence. I know now what I felt then. My conscious self realised it was an indication of something serious – my subconscious recognised the more sinister aspect of the symptom. I didn't fully grasp it then, but it was to be the first of many blows that would come thick and fast over the coming days. It was that first punch to the nose; the one that stings, then hurts, and begins the numbing process of an almighty beating, the last few blows of which, when on the floor unconscious, one is hardly aware.

She was seeing fine yesterday! And today she can barely make out a finger when I am holding it ten centimetres from her face. I feel like screaming. I feel sick to the core.

## 3) Day 1 – 7:18am, Friday 5th April 2013

I glance over at Vanessa as soon as I hear Millie say she can only see brown from one eye. It's serious and we know it. I am just amazed at the lack of panic in Millie, and start wondering how long the condition in her right eye has been there for. In time, I find out that children often don't notice if one of their eyes deteriorates in functionality. They compensate. They make do. They don't complain, or perhaps they're apprehensive about complaining, fearing it might be something they have done. It could be guilt holding them back.

Sore grief assails me at seeing Millie at that moment, there, sitting on our sofa, alone, waiting to go up to London, blind in one eye, and (as I would discover the next day) nearly blind in the other. I pick myself up. I realise this is just the beginning and that I have to see the day through. I have to act quickly. I have to get on. I'm afraid. I'm confused. I'm lost. The adrenaline has started pumping and I can feel it.

I need to leave for London. I need to cross the English countryside, my river of Acheron, and have my meeting with Millie's paediatrician.

# INTO THE DREAD ABYSS

*4) Day 1 – 7:40am, Friday 5th April 2013*

Millie and I catch the 7:40am train to Charing Cross. We had contemplated taking Millie straight to A&E (that again!) following our discovery of lack of vision but, on balance, felt that one more hour on the train would probably not compromise the overall situation. It turned out to be the best decision we made on Millie's behalf and materially shaped the way in which she would be treated over the coming months.

Dr D had been Millie's paediatrician right from the start. He was the one who came to The Portland when she was born, to give her an initial birth assessment (it's been a while and I can't remember what they're called, but ironically she scored a ten – the top mark). And we had seen him on a regular basis for all three of our children (Ellie Rose and Luca Jack being the eldest and youngest respectively, aged nine and four – more on them later). In other words, we trust him implicitly. We still do.

Dr D is also the person we went to see when Millie started to develop an excessive thirst some twelve months ago, when she was six. Initially, because she was otherwise well, the favoured 'let's wait a bit and see' approach was adopted. A condition called diabetes insipidus was mentioned for the first time then but discarded because 'children with this disease are often really unwell'. We ruled out Type 1 diabetes, but the thirst continued and it became less and less manageable, especially at night. Whenever we went on holiday, Millie would become distressed about water, or rather, not finding any. We would find her wandering the hotel room at two in the morning looking for her fluid fix. So we went back to Dr D, and this time were referred to a specialist endocrinologist in Harley Street (the hormone doctor). An initial blood test was inconclusive with regards to diabetes insipidus. We needed to do a urine test at home under certain conditions. This was also inconclusive. We went back and forth for a good eight months. There were various consultations with Dr D, and then with the hormone doctor, as well as further tests and urine analysis. We were in the process of planning a further appointment with our endocrinologist when the vision loss happened.

Back on the train to London, I take out my iPad and start Googling 'sudden loss of vision' – 25.3 million hits in less time than it takes for my eye to blink (I think 0.18 seconds). I must Google that too some time: does Google take longer than the blink of an eye to return results for 'How long does it take for my eye to blink?' Anyway, this is broadly what I find (all, ironically, quite obscure):

- Retinal detachment
- Vitreous haemorrhage
- Retinal vein occlusion
- Retinal artery occlusion
- Wet age-related macular degeneration
- Anterior ischemic optic neuropathy
- Optic neuritis
- Cerebrovascular accident

I discard the obvious ones like retinal detachment (surely that must hurt; Millie has no pain), wet age-related macular degeneration (whatever that is – but it has the word 'age' in it, so even I can make that intellectual leap) and cerebrovascular accident (something to do with veins, the brain and an accident – so no, not that one). To be fair, I am none the wiser and can't even begin to second-guess what it might be. They all look pretty serious. I look at Millie and text my wife, 'Prepare for bad news – I have a feeling this won't be fixed by putting a plaster on it'.

We are running early for our appointment, so I try and buy some time. Vanessa suggests we should phone ahead, explain the loss of vision and see if we can be seen more quickly once we arrive.

I look at Millie again – it's hard to describe the immense feeling of pain that fills every cell of your body when you look at your daughter, an innocent seven-year-old girl, entering limbo, probably lost in terrifying thoughts, not able to see and wondering what the hell is going on.

*5) Day 1 – 8:40am, Friday 5th April 2013*

We arrive at Charing Cross. I am now carrying Millie everywhere as it's clear she can't see. I try the finger test in the taxi, somehow hoping to observe some improvement – how desperately naïve parents can be. She moves her head to one side, gets it wrong most of the time and still says she can't see from her right eye. She's also getting fed up with me asking, so I stop. It's not going to improve her eyesight, it's just going to worry her more.

Our appointment is at 10am and we are there in plenty of time. I register with Dr D's secretary who tells me my wife has phoned ahead, but I don't sense any urgency in her tone. In any case, Dr D can see us pretty much straight away. I explain the situation to him (but without panic in my voice – maybe that's what initially confuses him). He looks at Millie, looks in her eyes, weighs her and listens to her chest. He asks me about the drinking and I say it's still the same but that we are seeing the hormone doctor soon. Dr D suggests it may be worthwhile doing a brain scan at some point (the first time it's been mentioned since the whole drinking thing started). But all in all, he says he's happy with Mille: "A bit of blurry vision is possibly tiredness, she seems well and let's keep in touch to review progress".

It takes me a good few seconds to clear my thoughts and for my brain to register what he's just said. Maybe the vision loss is not that serious after all? Did he actually hear me when I said it? Maybe I didn't explain it very well. Eventually I repeat the obvious: "Dr D, what about the fact that she can't see from her right eye *at all*? She says she can only see brown." His expression changes – and from that point on so does my world and that of my family. *Fuck*. It's serious.

He arranges an urgent MRI scan across the road at The Portland Hospital and sends me off, telling me to come back afterwards. I know the hospital well. All three of my children were born there. My eldest had her adenoids removed there and my youngest had a minor surgical intervention there when he was six months old. Now it's Millie's turn. This time it's an MRI scan.

A magnetic resonance imaging (MRI) scan uses strong magnetic fields and radio waves to take pictures of the brain or spine. It differs from a standard X-ray in that it produces a very detailed picture. It's also very noisy, as I would soon discover.

11

I'm still carrying Millie everywhere – she can barely make anything out. It's getting worse and worse, and every minute that passes feels like an eternity. We are finally called in and go through some consent forms. This includes answering a number of basic questions such as:

- Does she have a pacemaker? (Huh... No.)
- Does she have an artificial heart valve? (Huh... No!)
- Has she ever had surgery on her head? (Huh... No, though not for long as it turns out – but I didn't know that yet.)
- Does she have any metallic implants like joint replacements? (No.)
- Has she ever had metal in her eyes from welding or metalwork? (What? She's seven! No!)

I'm then asked to remove various items of clothing like my metal belt buckle, glasses, mobile phone and wallet with cards; anything that might be affected by the magnetic waves. They tell Millie and me that it will be very noisy, give me some earplugs, my daughter some earphones and ask her to choose a DVD (she can't see, but somehow it helps to pretend and at least she can listen to the sound). She goes for *Mary Poppins*. Good choice. Unfortunately for Millie, there will be no spoonfuls of sugar where she is heading over the coming months.

The MRI machine itself is a short tunnel, cream in colour, and open at both ends. Millie will lie on a motorised bed that is moved inside the scanner. She will enter the scanner head first with an open helmet to keep her head still (the bit we need to take pictures of). Millie will be able to see the TV screen with the help of a couple of well-placed small mirrors that eventually face towards a TV on the wall at the end of the scanner, with the picture upside down. MRI scans are normally painless and last about thirty minutes, but a contrast dye is often injected in order to create a clearer image. I explain all this to Millie, including the injection. She's not happy about it at all, though wasn't to know it was the first of many in the coming days.

I mentioned earlier that MRI scans are noisy. This is due to the electric current being turned on and off in whatever is moving around inside this magic tube. It alternates between a very loud tapping noise and what I can only describe as being in the middle of roadworks crammed with loud power tools.

It's loud for me (without earplugs as I want to hear what Millie hears – it somehow makes me feel more connected to her at this moment in time) but must be extra loud for her, like a furious invisible wind tossing her ceaselessly towards a much darker future.

When the MRI scan is finished, the nurses come in and I can sense a change in their approach, unable to hide the sadness I perceive in their eyes. I don't ask any questions, as I know they won't answer me. They tell me that the results are being sent to Dr D and I am to go back to see him as planned.

It's beginning to feel like a bad dream. I find it hard to focus, as if stuck in a merciless trance that won't let go of my soul.

Angst befalls me and everything inside me turns to black.


*6) Day 1 – 12:35pm, Friday 5th April 2013*


"Bad news, I'm afraid. It's a brain tumour," Dr D tells me. Time to wake up. I look outside. It's started to rain – like a storm of discoloured water.

# IN THE GRASS,
# THE SERPENT TRAINS

*7) Day 1 – 12:36pm, Friday 5th April 2013*

I try to remain composed. To be honest, I am so shocked I can barely think. Throughout the morning, one of my main objectives was to remain steady for Millie's sake. I was aware that children often look at parents for hints on how to behave and react when new information, that they might not understand very well, comes their way. I was determined to protect Millie, at least from a mental perspective (I knew I could do nothing to reverse or stop fast-growing cells).

"So, this lump in the brain…" I start tentatively.

"I think we should call it what it is," interrupts Dr D. "I'm going to call this a brain tumour." Brutal honesty. *Smack.* Another punch to the nose. My head is spinning. I can feel the heavy weight of responsibility slowly lowering on to my shoulders. There will be no sick notes available to get out of this. No magic plaster.

Dr D explains that we can't tell exactly what kind of tumour it is from the MRI scan. He is going to try and get in touch with one of his contacts at Great Ormond Street Hospital (GOSH, to those in the unfortunate position of knowing – or maybe it's what posh people say when they're told their daughter is very ill) to see if they might be able to see us today. It will take a couple of hours, so I should think about getting some lunch.

Millie and I cross the road to Pizza Express for 'wiggly pasta', one of her favourite meals. Before I go in, I call Vanessa. It is the hardest call I have made in my life so far. I know she is going to hurt. I know the words I'm about to deliberately utter will cause her immense suffering. I will be delivering news that will take her from a state of blissful ignorance to knowing her seven-year-old daughter has a brain tumour that may well end her life. But just as I deserved it earlier from Dr D, she deserves brutal honesty from me now.

I take a deep breath and ring Vanessa's number. She picks up; a degree of inquisitive apprehension in her voice. "It's a brain tumour," I say. I tell her the broad outline of the plan – which, at this stage, is nothing more than to wait two hours while Dr D gets in touch with his colleague at GOSH.

Millie orders her favourite and I order an American Hot Leggera, the one with the hole in the middle. Millie's hearty appetite shows she has no idea what's going on. I try my level best to keep it that way, though I know at some point I will have to explain some very unpleasant events that are likely to occur in the next few days.

At this stage, I have no idea what those might be, but one thing is certain: I fully appreciate my actions and decisions over the next two days may well define the rest of her life. For the first time since 7:12am, my senses begin to sharpen. My heartbeat slows and the world around me gradually begins to readjust to the right level of focus. Later that day, and for the next three days, as the nature of Millie's condition unfolds, something inexplicable happens – panic slowly oozes out and makes way for a sense of firmness, commitment and resolve I have never experienced before.

15

Time to go back to Dr D's consulting room. We cross the road again, Millie in my arms. I stop in front of the glass-fronted entrance and look up at the sky. 234 Great Portland Street stands in front of me, a lofty tower into which I now need to go and meet with destiny.

*8) Day 1 – 2:15pm, Friday 5th April 2013*

Still no news from GOSH – we wait outside Dr D's consulting rooms. Millie sits next to me, her eyes shut. She has stopped going anywhere in the room on her own other than a tentative attempt at reaching the water dispenser. Her suspected diabetes insipidus, unremorseful of her lack of vision, continues to drive her to sources of water when thirst materialises.

Still no news. We go for a coffee and hot chocolate at Pret a Manger next door (where Millie opens the first of many bags of popcorn). Still no news. We wait. And wait and wait. All this waiting time allows me to regroup and think what might become of us over the next few hours, days and months. The truth is I don't know. Uncertainty will become the dominant theme of the next few weeks, so I'd better get used to it. I take the opportunity to scan emails on my BlackBerry and send a couple of messages to my two fellow directors saying that I cannot deal with any work matters this afternoon and would be in touch later in the day to give them a full debrief. They still don't know what is happening.

Finally, Dr D calls us in. He holds a DVD of the MRI scan. He confirms he has been able to contact one of the neurosurgeons at GOSH and that I am to go to the hospital's Koala Ward and hand deliver the disc for the urgent attention of a Mr J. What I didn't realise until much later was the degree of effort being undertaken behind the scenes to move as quickly as possible in an attempt to stop Millie's gradual visual decline. He also prescribes a heavy dose of a steroid called dexamethasone, which is often used to reduce swelling. (He thinks the tumour, or lesions caused by it, might be putting pressure on the optic nerves; hence the loss of vision. Dexamethosone might help in easing that pressure.) Increased appetite is a common side effect of the drug, and many a bag of popcorn would perish over the next forty-eight hours as a result of Millie's ferocious hunger. He wishes me luck, asks me to keep him up to date and says he will get in touch later in the day to confirm the next steps with regards to GOSH admission. I register none of it.

Millie and I go to the pharmacy across the road, buy and administer the steroid together with another pill to protect the lining of her stomach. One of the side effects of the steroid is to irritate the stomach wall. An unfortunate irony: a drug that has the side effect of making you hungry also diminishes the ability of your stomach to cope with the food you eat.

We hop in a cab and I ask to go to GOSH. On arrival, I look for Koala Ward. Koala Ward cares for children within clinical specialties including neurology, telemetry (measuring brain electrical activity), craniofacial (treatment of certain congenital malformations of the face and skull) and neurosurgery (unbeknown to me then, the one Millie was going to need). The ward was easy to find. Less easy was walking through a ward where the patients are children afflicted by various cranial malformations and suffering from the aftermath of materially invasive operations – some children, many of whom were younger than Millie, had mini steel face scaffolds protruding from their heads.

I haven't spent much time in hospitals either for myself or for my loved ones, and was acutely aware that rapid adjustment needed to take place if I were to be any use to Millie May. It was perhaps the first and only time I felt a sense of disbelief about it all. The first and only time I felt detached from my own body, suspended in a state of incredulity and not quite conceiving this was actually happening to me, to us as a family, to Millie.

I hand over the DVD at reception, making sure they understand the gravity and urgency of the situation. I leave, trusting that the nurse would, in good faith, do her job and give the disc to Mr J.

My mind goes back over the events of today, and over the likely next steps. I'm not sure what those will be. Admission to GOSH is not at the forefront of my mind. It should be, but then what's happened has been so astronomically overwhelming that I can't be too hard on myself for lacking certainty as to what my focus and short-term objectives ought to be at each step of this, as yet undefined, road. I had heard of GOSH, of course: a centre of worldwide excellence, renowned for its dedication to curing children. Until now it had been a distant concept – a mythical city, whose stories I had read in newspapers or watched on documentaries. It was now a possibility that Millie would be admitted, though I wasn't sure of it yet. Will the demons refuse us entrance? It's still difficult to tell. Besides, I don't quite yet realise the importance of being admitted to GOSH. Much of the time that elapses does so without the benefit of an overall end game, the nature of which will only later become clearer.

Time to go back home. We catch a train back to Tunbridge Wells – Millie is exhausted; it's close to 7pm.


*9) Day 1 – 8:15pm, Friday 5th April 2013*

Vanessa has had the good judgment to send our other two

children to stay with Mama (pronounced Mah-Mah) – her mother. Vanessa's parents live approximately 500 yards away from our house – a blessing, as it will turn out to be. I had lived in London for the best part of sixteen years, but after our third child was born, it became too difficult and too congested for a family of five. So, after considering a few options, we settled for a little village just outside Tunbridge Wells, and right next to the church we had married in some seven years prior. It also felt a natural decision in the context of my own first move to England aged sixteen. I'm an Italian national (Italian parents) and, having been brought up in the South of France, I finished my education at a nearby school in Kent, very close to Tunbridge Wells.

Had I played rugby or football at school, no doubt I would have played against many of the schools in and around Royal Tunbridge Wells (I didn't – my main sport at school, an early indication of my general lack of ambition in life, was table tennis). We also happened to be aware of a very good school where Vanessa's brother had gone when he was young. All in all, the little East Sussex village offered both the security and sense of community that Vanessa required, especially as I was still working in London when we moved, so likely to regularly spend time away from home. It was close to her parents and sister, and she was very familiar with the area, having lived there most of her life. Those were happy days. Back to black.

So Ness (Vanessa, Ness, Nessy – depending on the mood and whether or not we've had an argument in the previous five minutes) had sent Ellie and Luca to Mama's. They would end up staying there for the next two weeks. Two weeks that would turn out to be the most intense and brutal two weeks of our lives so far.

The phone rings. Ness picks it up. It's Dr D. He confirms

that we should go to GOSH tomorrow morning at 10am for 'further tests' in view of being admitted as soon as possible, probably at some point the following week (today being Friday). I write an email to my co-directors to let them know. Reading it again as I write this diary reveals how unprepared I was for what was to come, and the degree of uncertainty that one feels during these unfamiliar situations. A later email to update my friends will expose the darkness that had beset as a result of the fuller diagnosis and, in particular, over the doubtful recovery of Millie's vision.

So, after a day spent in London, this is what we knew (or, as it turns out, what we didn't know):

- It was a brain tumour (Yep. That's right. A fucking brain tumour.)
- I knew nothing of brain tumours (why should I?), so I didn't know how serious it was. Obviously, I knew it was serious, but *how* serious, I did not know.
- I didn't know if it was cancer or a benign lump.
- I didn't know what kind of treatment or procedure it would require.
- I didn't know how long it would take to cure, and over how many different stages.
- I didn't know when and if we would be admitted somewhere.
- I didn't know if Millie would ever be the same again.
- I didn't know if she would regain her sight.
- I didn't know if she would die soon – though clearly, it had become a very real possibility that I couldn't even begin to process.

Here's what I did know. I knew I didn't know enough. I knew

that 'real-life' problem situations are always initially undefined, messy and without boundaries. I have always been able to accept that whenever a new situation in life presents itself, or when I am about to start learning a new topic or concept, it takes time and effort to adjust. Gradually boundaries begin to appear, fog lifts and clarity slowly but surely materialises. I recognise that by breaking big problems into smaller ones, it is easier to resolve them. Although the nature of this differed on an astronomical scale, I had to face it in the same way I had faced problems in the past.

It's getting late. Millie had no difficulty going to sleep. Ness and I don't talk much, we get into bed and try as much as we can to clear our heads of the disconsolate gloom that has taken residence in the very core of our beings.

Sadness raids my spirit and kills a little bit of me in the process. It won't be the last time something in me dies over the next couple of months.

# BETWEEN THE WALLS AND
# THE TORMENTED SOULS

*10) Day 2 – 6:23am, Saturday 6th April 2013*

Like the condemned who have knowledge of future things, but are ignorant of what is happening at present, it takes me a few seconds for the events of the previous day to come back to me when I first wake. Millie has had an adequate night, though with her eyesight now almost down to zero, it's no wonder she hasn't moved from her bed. I need to carry her downstairs for breakfast. She can barely see, though nonetheless seems in good spirits. Children are amazing creatures in this respect, and this characteristic would hold true for the remainder of her future treatment. Unlike adults, children very rarely feel sorry for themselves. They accept their illness with stoic indifference and just get on with it. It still breaks your heart to see them suffer in blissful ignorance of the tragic affliction befalling them. But at least to some degree they don't know any better. Or rather, they only extrapolate from the behaviour of adults around them, and in particular (and so it should be) their parents.

Vanessa and I make a deliberate decision to adopt a 'serious-yet-composed' disposition to protect Millie from the sinister nature of her illness and, more importantly perhaps, the discomfort she will have to endure in order to get better and be cured. We know little (well, nothing) at this stage of the three nine-hour brain operations, the four months of gruelling chemotherapy at GOSH and the thirty sessions of proton beam therapy she will undergo at a specialist centre in the USA in September and October later this year. And just as well, actually.

So we set off to London once again, earlier than we needed. We know we can't be late for our 10am appointment at GOSH. The train journey is a sad one; Millie is now very much within herself, not able to see anything (or next to nothing). It seems a good time to let people know. Vanessa's family knows by necessity, as we left Ellie and Luca to stay last night. I still haven't told my parents or my sister. I've already had to break the news once to Ness. I'm not looking forward to doing it again.

My sister M and I haven't seen much of each other over the past eight years. In fact, I've probably seen her twice in the past two years, and only as a result of a Christmas family lunch organised by my mother, in an attempt to reduce the rift that time has widened between the pair of us. There are probably reasons why we don't talk, but whatever they are, they are all outside the scope of this diary, so I will leave out any attempt at analysis. Be that as it may, I feel the need to let M know about Millie and about what is happening. I know I will have to tell my parents, and as they are getting older, this piece of news is going to be hard on them. I feel M deserves a say on how I will do that, and also forewarning of it. They are her parents too. I had sent a brief message earlier in the day to establish if she was receiving emails (she was on holiday), which she was (receiving emails that is). So I send her one from the train explaining the situation:

*Hi,*

*We found out yesterday that Millie has a brain tumour. We are going back to London for further tests this morning. We don't know the details yet or possible prognosis but it's clearly very serious, whatever it turns out to be. It is very likely that she will be admitted to Great Ormond Street Hospital in the next few days.*

*I have not told Mum and Dad yet as they are old and in poor health, and I'm not sure how they will react to the news. But clearly they need to know. So it would be good to talk and have your thoughts, as at the moment my only focus is Millie and am unlikely to have time to deal with any Mum and Dad-type events.*

*I will try and call you on your mobile later today. Am on the train to Great Ormond Street Hospital at the moment to meet the neurosurgeon and establish a plan. Hopefully I'll know more about the type of tumour and likely sequence of events later today.*

*All in all, a very bad week.*
*M*

The tone is calm – I know I cannot change what Millie has, or the treatment that will be required to cure her. All I know is that Ness and I need to act as the custodians of her health and wellbeing by making sure we are organised and can act with focus and resolve. 'Establish plan', 'sequence of events', 'knowing the details'. This is the language of project management. I sense that our roles will be that of facilitators, making sure we are in the right place at the right time, and alongside Millie throughout. I realise it's going to be hard, but somehow I feel up to the task. This morning's task is to get her to GOSH.

M's response following the email is immediate and heartfelt. She calls me on my mobile and I update her as best I can. For the first time since the diagnosis, I feel like crying and it's hard to fight back the tears as I explain the situation to my sister.

## 11) Day 2 – 9:12am, Saturday 6th April 2013

We arrive at Koala Ward with plenty of time to spare, and are asked to wait in the reception area. We are told that Mr J, the lead neurosurgeon, and his team will come and talk to us shortly. At this stage, we are still completely clueless as to what awaits us. We are very much reactive and only just starting to smell the fetid steam that rises from the abyss into which we will shortly be thrown 'good and proper'. Millie has started her second bag of popcorn, probably as a result of boredom, not being able to see, and the steroid she has been taking since yesterday afternoon.

Mr J and his team of three or four finally arrive and he sits down in front of us. He is a softly spoken gentleman of Kashmiri descent. Despite our infinite anguish, we like him immediately. A good thing, as we would find out shortly, because he is the one who will, tomorrow morning, cut out a piece of Millie's skull to access a tumour set deep in her brain. He asks us to summarise the events of the last couple of days, which we do as best we can.

For the first time since diagnosis, we are finally told what Millie has. Mr J believes, on seeing the MRI scan, that Millie has a craniopharyngioma, a type of brain tumour derived from pituitary gland embryonic tissue that occurs most commonly in children. It's rare, it's benign and is probably surgically accessible, though in a sensitive spot of the brain. (I thought every part of the brain would be a pretty sensitive spot... It's also not what Millie has, as we would later find out, so don't Google the term just yet, as I did that morning.)

The plan for the day is twofold, says Mr J. Firstly, Millie needs a number of additional tests, including an eye examination at Moorfields Eye Hospital and a CT scan to confirm initial diagnosis. CT, as many of the nurses I asked didn't know, stands for 'computerised tomography', and is also known as a CAT scan. It uses X-rays and a computer to create detailed images of the inside of, in Millie's case, the brain. *Tomo* being Greek for 'section'. The CT scan provides a different level of detail to the MRI scan, which will be needed should we decide to operate.

This brings me to the 'secondly'. Secondly, time has never been more against us as it is today, and Millie's eyesight is deteriorating with every revolution of the second's hand. She can see next to nothing at the moment, so it is of critical importance to establish a precise diagnosis to see how quickly and *whether* we can operate. Also, whether the operation can improve matters as far as Millie's vision is concerned.

A minute feels like an eternity under the current circumstances, but the CT scan won't happen until later this afternoon, as one of the machines is broken. So we should start the admission process, be allocated a room and get a few of the more minor tests out of the way. These are weight, height and blood tests. A needle in the arm seems minor but painful nonetheless if you are seven, scared and blind. Luckily, Millie would not have to suffer on that front for much longer but she was still going to be pricked a few times over the

26

coming days. We are also told that we will not be going home – and this, paradoxically, reassures us.

This seems the right time to give my parents the heads up. I know it will upset them. I call my mother and update her; we don't know much at the moment but I promise to keep her informed as the day progresses.

That's it, everyone in our respective families now knows. We feel less alone.

## 12) Day 2 – 11:32am, Saturday 6th April 2013

We get confirmation that Moorfields is aware of our situation and we should get there as soon as possible to be seen by one of the consultants.

We leave Koala Ward, jump in a taxi and get to Moorfields. It is the oldest (and looks it) and largest eye hospital in the world, internationally renowned for its comprehensive clinical and research activities. The hospital is a major international care and training centre in ophthalmology (eye stuff), and apparently over half of all ophthalmologists in the UK have received specialist training at the hospital. The waiting room is full of people with eye problems, ranging from slight redness to conditions that look pretty awful.

We are seen very quickly by the consultant, who runs some basic tests. Millie is made to stand at one end of the corridor and is asked to look at pictures of varying size, at certain distances. She does pretty poorly and seems to be moving her head from side to side as if she were only able to see from a certain angle. The consultant ophthalmologist (senior eye doctor) then looks at her optic nerve and detects some signs of life. It's still pink but not healthy; at least it's not white though

– a bad thing, apparently. He confirms Millie is suffering from what he believes to be optic nerve compression, with very little or no perception of light in the right eye and 6/60 in the left. This means she can see at six metres away what a normal person can see sixty metres away – or ten times less than a normal person. I believe he also indicates that she has some peripheral temporal vision left, but nothing on the nasal side.

The eye doctor calls the lead consultant on duty to discuss the next steps (It's a Saturday. So this is a phone call). All in all, they feel that whatever needs to be done can wait till Monday, for reasons I am as yet unclear about. Time has never been more of the essence as it was on that day and thankfully, and I still don't know why, I understood that and realised these guys were not going to make the critical decision to try and save her eyesight. Odd perhaps, given Moorfields is a hospital specialising in eye care. You would have thought they would be slightly more anxious to try and preserve as much of Millie's vision as possible. Not so.

I instinctively knew I had to get her back to Koala Ward as quickly as possible. I think I recognised that the neurosurgeon and his team felt an emergency operation was required in order to preserve some vision – and I liked that scenario better, even if it meant Millie having to go under the knife in the most traumatic way. Moorfields couldn't help us any more, there was no point in hanging around, so I ask for the summary notes to take with us; and off we go, back to GOSH.

Despair does not even begin to describe how we feel at this moment in time. As we travel back in the taxi, this is where I think we are:

- Millie is now significantly visually impaired. For all intents and purposes, she is blind and may never recover her sight.

- Every minute that goes by she loses further vision, or rather, potential to improve in the future.
- She has a brain tumour that, whilst benign (or so we think), is in a tricky position to operate on.
- We have no idea how to resolve this situation. We have no idea what will unfold over the next twenty-four hours.

Things surely can't get any worse... Unfortunately for Millie and for us, they do. Travelling back to GOSH in that taxi, we were not to know that we had yet to cross our river of blood, and we did not know if fate would afford us safe passage to the other side.

# A FOREST, WHERE NO
# TRACK OF STEPS HAD
# WORN A WAY

*13) Day 2 – 3:17pm, Saturday 6th April 2013*

We arrive back at GOSH and are asked to wait in the reception area. Millie has perked up a little. The steroid she has been taking since yesterday may well be having an effect on the swelling and easing the pressure on her optic nerve. Besides eating popcorn as if her life depended on it, she has gained enough confidence to skip between Vanessa and me, at either end of the reception area. She is still tilting her head, can broadly see in the direction she wishes to go, and her legs have remained unimpaired by the trauma so far. It's a sorry sight to see her try so hard to show us she is normal, this child of ours, who was well two days ago, and is now on the verge of a precipice, unaware of her inescapable fall.

Fall she will. What we don't know is if she will survive the landing. We try to keep up appearances by encouraging her and letting her know how well she's doing.

Time for our CAT scan – another painless, magical piece of equipment; very similar to an MRI scan. At least Millie is now used to it, and we know she can lie still.

We still don't know if the operation will be taking place tomorrow or at some point the following week. To be honest, lack of knowledge (or rather foresight) is the theme of the day, and will be so over the next fortnight. It's a difficult situation compounded by the stress and doubly compounded by the fact it's all very new to us. Oh yeah, and our daughter is now blind and has a tumour, which we will later be told is actually cancer. We know that while our empathy is astronomical, she is the one that will have to endure it and, perhaps more pointedly, endure the cure which often makes you feel significantly worse than the illness itself (in the short term, definitely; in the long term, possibly). More on that lovely stuff later on.

At the moment, we feel overwhelmed by events, but perhaps more prevalent is the feeling of doubt and whether we are doing the right thing for Millie. We don't know GOSH, we don't know Mr J and his team, we don't really understand the clinical nature of what she has, and we don't know the alternatives. Over the coming days, we will need to give consent to opening up our daughter's head, risking greater health consequences, and making her significantly worse before she gets a bit better (maybe, perhaps, possibly). The multitude of consent forms that we, her parents, will have to sign make it quite clear. And all of this goes against the protective instincts one has as a parent, of course.

My own natural disposition for rational behaviour (some say, wrongly, indifferent) will probably help Millie's cause over the next few days, and a new-found rational streak to Vanessa's character emerges as we solidify the trust we have in each other when making tough decisions about our children.

There is a big difference between choosing a school, for example, and choosing for your seven-year-old to have a brain operation. Over the next seventy-two hours, we get quite good at being rational and leaving our emotions in check to try and act in Millie's best interests in the most harrowing of circumstances. All of this may well be an illusion, of course. We are probably made to feel like we are given choices, like a nine-year-old made to choose between pre-selected schools. It may be a well-orchestrated strategy by the medical profession who use a careful balance of limiting choices and gradual disclosure. More on gradual disclosure later on, by the way. We discover the true meaning of it as the next few days unfold.

For the moment, we were treading fearfully on an uncertain path, in a dark forest, where no track of steps had worn a way; or at least, not by our own steps.

*14) Day 2 – 6:17pm, Saturday 6th April 2013*

The quiet room in Koala Ward is a small consulting room, near the entrance of the ward. I suspect it has witnessed anguish of the deepest kind over the years, as it is here that one is usually taken to be told of the unfolding events linked to your child's diagnosis (usually significant and severe in this ward). It is to this room we are now taken for a talk with one of the neurosurgeons. Like the condemned, we reticently go in with Millie, who is distracted by Maria, one of the nurses.

Maria: an apt name for a young senior nurse who would show me, us as a family and Millie, compassion and kindness on a most overwhelming scale. This level of care, as we would learn, is duplicated with regular consistency among the nurses in Koala Ward, but it is Maria who I will remember the most. She made a difference on that dark day. She brought a glimmer of candlelight to an otherwise dark, tormented soul. Later that evening, Maria asked me about my other two children, and for the first time since the diagnosis, I cried. She took me aside into an empty room to help me gather my thoughts. Her humanity, which came naturally to her, gave me strength that evening. It restored my faculty for composure. I am grateful to you, Maria. I will remember you always. You touched my heart and I wish you well. You were grace in the most unexpected place, at the most unexpected time.

Back in the quiet room, we are shown the CT and MRI pictures of Millie's tumour for the first time on a computer screen. It is confirmed to most likely be a craniopharyngioma (a benign tumour about the size of a golf ball), and we have some options (yeah, right!) to consider:

- Do nothing for the time being. What Millie has is a threat to her life, but the *urgency* is more to do with her eyesight, or lack of it.
- Operate for the sole objective of *preserving* her eyesight.

'Preserving' hits me like a fast-moving train. At this stage, there is no language to suggest that Millie's eyesight will return or improve. In fact, it may well get worse as a result of the intervention, which she may or may not have. Fuck, fuck, fuck and fuck. I repeat my thoughts in disbelief: the objective of the operation, if she has one, is to try and *preserve* the little vision she has left. If she can have one in the next twenty-four hours! It's Sunday tomorrow, so GOSH only has one surgical operating room available with already a full operating schedule (they're busy with other children as equally in need as Millie) but they are trying their level best to gather a team in order to open the second room.

It becomes clear to us that the lead neurosurgeon and his

number two currently talking to us believe an urgent operation is the best (and only) choice. And they are doing their utmost to come into work on a Sunday to undertake an eight-hour operation on my daughter. Wow! I've never felt that way about completing a spreadsheet. It blows my mind, and not for the first time. I am grateful to these people, to whom Millie is a complete stranger, and who always *put the child first and always,* because they believe it is the right thing to do. They are the living, breathing embodiment of that famous tag line. I feel like kissing everyone in this place. But I restrict myself to just letting them know that.

I soon change my mind about kissing when the neurosurgeon briefly explains the risks associated with the operation and asks me to sign a consent form ('It's not my fault if it goes wrong, Guv' of hospitals the world over). Millie will undergo a bicoronal, subfrontal craniotomy and debulking of suprasellar abnormality. In plain English, they are going to cut her head open from ear to ear and remove enough of the tumour located in the vicinity of the hypothalamus and pituitary gland to let the optic nerve breathe a little better.

It's easy to be lulled and underestimate the severity of an operation when you hear it described in the language of the medical profession. Let me explain. More specifically, this is what my lovely seven-year-old daughter will have done to her after they put her to sleep (maybe, possibly, perhaps tomorrow morning, but no one can tell us with any certainty): an incision will be made from one ear to the other, about half an inch from where her hairline starts. Her scalp will then be pulled back across her face to expose most of her forehead. At which point, a little bone window will be cut out by drilling four holes, one at each corner of the window, and then joined up by dragging the drill from one hole to the other. With the brain thus exposed, the surgeon will be free to roam and find

34

the bulk of the tumour and chip away at it a tiny piece at a time in order to relieve pressure on the optic nerve (for vision 'preservation' – a grand word for the little that remains…), get enough of the tumorous mass to perform a histological analysis, and decompress the mass *if* he can. Oh, and while he is there, he might as well take as much out as possible without compromising the surrounding tissue, which is mostly made up of brain matter.

All of this, of course, is not without risks ('serious or frequently occurring' as stated on the consent form), the main ones being:

- Infection: Okay, I can probably live with that one.
- Bleeding and stroke: a little less pleasant.
- CSF Leak (CSF standing for 'cerebrospinal fluid'. The skull is reinforced by three strata of protective tissue known as the meninges, in between which is a liquid called cerebrovascular fluid, acting as a special shock-proof layer): I've no idea if this is serious but it certainly doesn't sound good.
- Risk of life: I think one of the neurosurgeons inadvertently omitted the words 'loss of' before the word 'life', but I get the gist and don't feel it's the right time to be pedantic; surely that's enough? Are there any more…? Oh yes, there are.
- Endocrine issues: that's it, but massive in itself as I'll explain at length later on. They would have needed a whole day to list and explain the endocrine issues, and there's no time.

That's it. Ah, no. Wait! Just before the operation, when it eventually goes ahead, and after the worst conversation Vanessa and I have ever had, the lead neurosurgeon adds a few more to the form, including: hypothalamic disturbances (like endocrine issues, this one is vast too), and one last one I cannot read, but at this stage it's very much 'in for a penny, in for a pound', so it doesn't really matter anymore.

Of all the risks, the one that may affect Millie for the longest, in a way we cannot even begin to grasp, is the endocrine disruption to the hormones. The pituitary gland is effectively the master gland as it controls and regulates most, if not all, of the hormones secreted by various organs in the body throughout life.

This collection of chemical-releasing cells, in an area not bigger than a pea, may well end up tormenting Millie like incessant flakes of fire eternally showering down upon her.


*15) Day 2 – 7:20pm, Saturday 6th April 2013*

We finally move into our room to settle for the night, and are told that while we don't know for certain if Millie will be operated on in the morning, we should prepare as if she were. So she's to be nil by mouth for a certain number of hours before the operation. Not eat or drink? She has excessive uncontrollable thirst because of her probable diabetes insipidus, and she's on a steroid that causes excessive and uncontrollable hunger. Sometimes, you *really* are kicked when you're down.

It's dark. Figuratively, literally, metaphorically, symbolically and in every which way you look at it. I have always found the evenings more difficult, with greater propensity for the blues. It's at night, when I'm alone with my thoughts, that gloom rises and I think of nothing but the worst. Besides the imminent operation and brain tumour, here's what I read up on endocrine and hypothalamic issues, and craniopharyngiomas more generally (though remember reader, this is *not* what Millie actually has. It's what they think she has based on the CT and MRI scans. To be fair, whatever she has, these issues hold as they relate more to the region of the brain where the growth lies, than the nature of the growth itself). I just don't know if I would refer to these potentially life-changing cataclysmic events as 'issues':

- If the tumour compresses the pituitary gland or pituitary stalk, it can cause the following: stunted growth (tick! Ahhh! Now that you mention it, Millie has been on the small side of late when compared to her peers); delayed puberty; loss of normal menstrual function; loss of sexual desire; increased sensitivity to cold (tick to the last one!); fatigue; constipation (tick, tick!); dry skin; nausea; low blood pressure; depression; diabetes insipidus (aha! Tick!); increased prolactin levels; and milky discharge from the breasts (euh! No! Not yet!).
- If the tumour compresses the optic nerves or optic chiasm, it can cause the following: blurred vision (tick!); decreased visual field (tick!); blindness (increasingly… tick!).
- If the tumour compresses the hypothalamus, it can cause the following: obesity (Millie's weight would eventually become an issue as the treatment progresses), increased drowsiness, body temperature regulation abnormalities, diabetes insipidus, personality changes, headache, confusion, vomiting.

And that's just the tumour, folks! Its removal has the following lovely risks attached to it: vision loss; seizures; hypothalamic injury (see risks above); morbid obesity; memory and behavioural problems; disturbance of sleep cycle and temperature regulation; and pituitary damage (see risks above).

This is not something that will resolve itself in a couple of weeks. This is going to be a long, hard slog. No wonder I feel gloomy.

As I fall asleep and tiredness takes hold of me, I replay the day and try to make sense of the information that has come our way from all the medical staff we have encountered – this troop of spirits, who will no doubt haunt my nights from now on.

We still don't know if the operation will happen, and we still don't know what the night will bring and how it will affect the remaining small parcels of light that are still travelling down Millie's optic nerves.

# THROUGH THE GROSS AND MURKY AIR, A SHAPE COMES SWIMMING UP

*16) Day 3 – 8:45am, Sunday 7th April 2013*

It is not until 8:45am that we finally get confirmation that they have managed to mobilise a team and Millie will be operated on by Mr J this morning, at around 10am. She is the first one in and Mr J will come and talk to us shortly (remember, the worst conversation Vanessa and I have ever had…).

Mr J, soft-spoken and calm, comes in and broadly covers what his number two told us the day before, but with a greater degree of brutality. He manages our expectations to such an extent we end up feeling that if Millie comes back at all from the operation, she will be blind, with severe endocrine dysfunction, and with a high risk of strokes and blood clots. Wallop – another kick in the stomach. By now we're on the metaphorical floor, knees bent, our hands on our heads, as if trying to limit the number of kicks that have come our way since yesterday.

We understand there is no choice; he believes it is the right course of action and we believe it is the right thing to do. "You are being very brave," he tells us, as if to try and make us feel better about ourselves and the situation.

"There's nothing brave about this", I reply. "Brave is when you have a choice, Mr J." I'm annoyed. I don't need mollycoddling. I don't need protection or reassurance from another grown-up. I'm an adult – just keep fucking kicking me and let's be done with it.

I glance over at Millie lying on her bed. I know she will go through hell over the coming weeks, and it's likely she will never be the same Millie again. Here we are, in Room 13, preparing for our seven-year-old daughter to be taken down to theatre, where she will undergo an operation that will last some seven or eight hours, the outcome of which is unknown. The degree of success, if any, is also unknown, but her suffering is a certainty. I need to start to readjust my own expectations on a time frame. This is not about today, tomorrow or next week. This will require sustained effort over a very long period of time.

Over the last two days we have tried, using age-appropriate language, to keep Millie informed as to what is happening to her. She has always preferred to know things and be told the truth, no matter how unpleasant, and be 'treated as a grown-up'. We sit down on her bed and explain that she is about to have an operation (she knew this was a possibility). She has to have this in order for her eyesight to get better and to remove a little ball of cells inside her brain that's making her sick. She will be asleep, so won't feel any pain, other than the injection required to go to sleep, but it will be over before she knows it. She will feel very poorly for a week after the operation, but Mummy and Daddy will be with her throughout. Millie seems to react relatively well to all this information but doesn't understand the more sinister aspect of her condition. Just as well, really.

We ask Millie how she wants to go down to the operating

theatre and she chooses to be carried by me. Even writing this is difficult. I can sense my tears rising as I feel the warmth of her body next to mine; this poor parcel of innocence, about to embark on the most traumatic voyage of her life. It hurts deep inside my heart, and in places I didn't know existed, to realise that this may be the last time I hold Millie in my arms. I have had her for seven years, seven beautiful years, and I have grown to love every single cell of her body. She is beautiful, and young, and bright and, as it turns out, she is very sick indeed.

We arrive at the operating theatre, or rather the vestibule adjacent to it, where Millie will be put to sleep. In unnecessarily laborious medical terms, this is where the anaesthesiologist will start transitioning her from the normal awake state to the sleepy state of aesthesia, also called induction. Millie opts for an injection in her arm while I hold her, not a single cry or complaint in sight, though she is clearly apprehensive – such a brave little thing. They tell me it will all happen quickly and within seconds her eyes roll back and she's departed. Throughout the process, we tell her we love her; we tell her we will be there when she wakes; we tell her all of this will soon be over. We tell her, despite knowledge to the contrary, that everything is going to be okay.

I place her gently on the small bed that will be used to take her into the operating theatre. We kiss her forehead, possibly for the last time, and leave the room, as the murky shadows of grief take residence in the viscera of our tormented souls.

The Millie we have known for seven years is dead. A new version may come back – we just don't know at this stage if and how closely related to the original she will be – or how long she will be with us for.

41

As we go back to our room Vanessa bursts into tears. I think it's what is generally referred to as crying your eyes out. Despair, disbelief and a sense of injustice, no doubt, are compounding her sense of grief. I try my best to console her, but this time there is nothing I can do to make Millie better. I tell her that we have each other, that we still have to think about Ellie and Luca, and that we will dedicate ourselves to making Millie better over the coming months.

The last remnants of horror escape my body. Nothing in the world matters other than the investment of time, effort and money we need to make in order to navigate the thorny road to recovery. I am aware I have other commitments such as my other two children and work, but for some reason, single-mindedness takes over and the sharpness of focus that started a couple of days ago increases to a level I have never experienced before. I *know* I will dedicate the next six months to holding Millie's hand throughout all that awaits. I *know* I will make the necessary sacrifices to free up my time in order to do so. I *know* other areas of my life may well suffer as a result, but I don't care. Something has taken over that will drive me through the gross and murky air of cancer (as we will soon discover Millie has) to an as yet uncertain conclusion. This new sense of resolve is not God, by the way, or some vague religious force (more on that fallacy later) – I can't put a name to it, as I have never felt it before. I'm sure every parent in a similar situation knows what I'm talking about. I'm reassured to feel this way, and that in itself gives me the strength I know I will require over the coming months.

The operation is likely to last anything from four to eight hours, we are told, and bar a tragic outcome, it is unlikely we would hear any updates from the operating theatre before the end. So we might as well try and keep our minds off it. I happen to have a small flat in London so we decide to go there and freshen up. Neither of us has showered since yesterday morning, and it will be good to leave GOSH for a few hours, despite our instincts to remain as close to Millie as possible. We leave the hospital, after giving our mobile phone numbers with the nurses, who, once again, have been incredible, and we take a taxi back to the flat.

My mind casts back over what has unfolded so violently over the last couple of days, and I am hit with the realisation that *it was cancer all along*: all the little symptoms Millie had over the last twelve months, the headaches, the thirst, the tendency to fatigue more quickly than her siblings, feeling the cold more than the average child. And while we went to see the right people at the right time, the outcome was inevitable. She was always going to end up in this place. As is often the case, but usually never recited in such a dramatic fashion, life's narrative only truly makes sense in retrospect. Cancer creeps up on you, and we can't beat ourselves up for what is happening to Millie. We later find out that some parents experience guilt when their child has cancer (for not discovering it sooner). Neither of us did – and whenever Vanessa attempted to attribute guilt to something she might have done (either during pregnancy, or later), I made sure she understood in the strongest possible terms that it was not our fault. In fact, I sensed that the 'fight' against cancer was going to be a marathon rather than a sprint, and our duty as parents was to expend energy in the most sensible, economical way. We needed to achieve the right balance between going through the processes necessary to make Millie better and ensuring we could go the distance. Feeling guilty was simply wasted energy.

Incidentally, the 'fight' against cancer is not a fight at all, and I have grown to loathe the belligerent nature of vocabulary used to describe the process of curing the disease (more on that later). Also I am neither religious nor do I allow myself the comfort of false pretences offered by alternative medicine and all who support it, those unscrupulous sellers of hope.

So, back at the flat, we wash, we change and we get a taxi back to GOSH. The mood is sombre, but both of us seem to be holding up adequately given the circumstances. The situation we are in is beyond our control, we understand that, and we understand the role we need to play. It's now 1pm, and there's no news from the operating theatre yet. The likelihood is that she'll be in for another couple of hours at least, so we take the opportunity to go for a bite to eat. Neither of us feels like it, but we haven't eaten anything since yesterday morning and are conscious our bodies need fuel to operate properly. There is a nice Pret a Manger opposite Russell Square tube station. It's close enough to the hospital for us to get back within five minutes should Millie unexpectedly come out of her operation early. We sit by the window with some food and drinks.

We go back over the last couple of days, and indeed the last couple of years, as it becomes clear Millie has had this for a long time. There is so much uncertainty about everything. And still more bad news to come. We realise we need to try and live in the moment, and we start adopting, in a very deliberate way, an attitude we will work hard on perfecting over the coming months. Professional golfers are familiar with it – it's called 'one shot at a time'. I guess it's the same in any sport, but golf is my hobby so I can relate to it better.

Broadly, professional golfers try to only think of their next shot, and ensure they execute it in order to give themselves the easiest possible next shot. They don't think much ahead of that;

they don't run away with their thoughts. They focus on the here and now, not on what they eventually hope to score when they finish the round – it's their philosophy. Golfers know that if they execute each and every shot in the best possible way, in the long term, they'll end up carding good scores overall, rather than bad ones. Focusing on the here and now means you are less likely to become overwhelmed by the enormity of the task ahead. You don't get distracted by others or by your surroundings. You focus on the task at hand and direct your energy into being the best you can be at completing it. You also avoid disappointment that way – it's one method to manage your own expectations. You don't run away with optimism, you keep that particular emotion in check by thinking only of the task you need to complete. It's particularly important, we feel, in a situation such as the one we are in, because there are so many variables and uncertainties that it's difficult to tangibly define an end game, a final objective of sorts. Besides, there probably isn't one. This is something we will have to manage for a long time yet.

2:35pm. We walk back to GOSH. No news yet, but we decide to wait in the reception area, where we had been the morning before, and where Millie was attempting to skip the previous evening. We sit and wait. We take the time to keep our respective families as up to date as possible. They deserve for the communication to be frequent, even if it's to tell them that we don't have any news.

We wait. And wait. And wait.


*18) Day 3 – 3:27pm Sunday 7th April 2013*

Mr J finally appears in the reception area. He comes to sit

next to us. It's an anxious moment. Our apprehension is easy to see, and he finally mutters: "It's gone very well." They were able to access the site and debulk the tumour to relieve pressure on the optic nerve. They took very little out, just enough to let the nerve breathe a little and hopefully try and preserve some of Millie's remaining vision. Overall, he is very happy with how the operation went, but is now 95% sure this thing is an astrocytoma, rather than a craniopharyngioma. An astrocytoma is a lump, but is classified as cancer as there are both benign and more aggressive types that spread throughout the brain. He doesn't tell us that though. In fact, I come away from the conversation thinking it was broadly similar to a craniopharyngioma, as he explains that the plan will remain pretty much the same. He also informs us that he's taken a sufficient amount for the histology to be performed and establish what the lump is once and for all. I sign the consent form for GOSH to send a sample of the tumour to be analysed.

Mr J tells us that Millie is in 'resus' (resuscitation) and quite confused. He needs us there straight away to see whether her sight is any better before swelling occurs around the eyes. He seems hopeful of a positive outcome. We follow him into resus, and finally see Millie (she's *alive!*), wriggling on the bed, tubes coming out of everywhere, like a ghost making low melancholy sounds. She immediately settles on hearing Vanessa's voice and asks for some water. Somewhat cruelly, Mr J asks us to put the bottle slightly out of reach to see if she can identify its location. It's clear she can't. Confused from the operation and the latent effect of the anaesthetic, or blind, or probably both, her outstretched hands desperately try to feel their way round the bed to find the bottle of water she has been promised. "Are you still hopeful with regards to her eyesight?" I ask.

Mr J seems flustered by the question, as if he wants to try and avoid answering it. "Difficult to tell. Let's see… Let's wait and see." That's it, I say to myself. She's blind.

# THENCE TO MY VIEW
# ANOTHER VALE APPEARED

*19) Day 3 – 4:46pm, Sunday 7th April 2013*

Millie calms down sufficiently and is stable enough to be brought
up to the high dependency unit (intensive care) in Koala Ward.
She will remain here for two to three days and be checked every
hour 24/7, until the doctors are satisfied she can be transferred to
a private room where she will be checked on less often (every
three hours). She has several tubes coming out of her, including:

- **A drip**. This is attached to a cannula on her left hand.
  Useful for blood transfusions, medicines and fluids until
  she is eating and drinking again.
- **Arterial line**. A tube into an artery in her ankle for taking
  blood samples and accurately measuring blood pressure.
  This will be very useful for the many blood samples
  required over the next few days to establish her
  endocrinological needs, without having to take blood the
  normal way, via a needle.
- **Drain**. The drain comes out of her wound and across the
  crown of her head. This is connected to a bag that is
  already gathering blood and tissue fluid from the operation.

- **Catheter**. A tube into her bladder so that her urine output can be measured (again, with her possible diagnosis of diabetes insipidus, this will be very useful).

Luckily, Millie has no need for a nasogastric tube for food at this stage (nor ever, thankfully). Still, four tubes coming out of your seven-year-old daughter in one go is something that takes a bit of time to adjust to.

Overall, despite our knowledge of her broader condition, she still looks like Millie May. Sure, she has a scar running from one ear to the other, about an inch inside of her hairline, but she's not particularly swollen (yet…). I was expecting the kind of face you see on cosmetic surgery programmes, where the woman comes out black and blue and looking like she's gone ten rounds with Mike Tyson. Not so with Millie. We are told that some swelling of the eyes will slowly occur over the next two days.

The high dependency ward has four beds, one in each corner of the room and a nurse monitoring each of the four patients every hour. There are two to four nurses, along with student nurses, at any given time, and all are incredible, extraordinary people in every way. They are kind, compassionate and understanding of our situation, without ever being patronising or in any way betraying the fact that for them, this, what we're going through, is part of their daily work routine. I will always remember the nurses in Koala Ward for the enormous capacity they have for humanity and the wellbeing of their fellow human beings. Clearly, it is their job to look after ill children, but still, I think they are head and shoulders above what we have experienced in other hospitals so far – and your names, Maria, Vanessa, Chloe and Jesse, in particular, will remain forever engraved on the deepest parts of my heart. In our darkest moments, you have made *all* the difference.

And the nurses were not the only people who would show us compassion on a scale most overwhelming. While I would not wish it on anyone, Millie's cancer was, in a sense, a gift. It revealed a side to human nature we seldom encounter during our brief moment in the sun, brainwashed by the media into thinking most strangers are paedophiles, murderers or rapists. On those rare occasions when we are forced to interact, by necessity, with people we don't know, we are often surprised by the kindness and generosity of those outside our immediate network of friends and family.

It's getting late. Millie is stable but somewhat sleepy, as she is on morphine as pain relief. With a nod and a wink, we are told that both my wife and I can stay the night, but one of us needs to go into one of the empty rooms across the ward. Being the better sleeper, I send Vanessa away to try and have as much of a restful night as possible. I prepare myself for some degree of sleep deprivation over the coming days, though having had three children (one with reflux up to the age of nine months), I am fully prepared for a few very short and interrupted nights.

Overcoming the operation was a major rock face to have climbed. Several more ascents were going to be required, some of which I could vaguely perceive, others yet too distant and remote for me to fully grasp their difficulty. One shot at a time, I tell myself. One shot at a time.


*20) Day 4 – 1:15am, Monday 8th April 2013*

The reclining chair made available for the parent who elects to stay in the high dependency unit is not particularly comfortable – but then I have slept in far less comfortable places in my life, and I have never been a particularly fussy sleeper. Still, the night is not without its incidents, though unexpectedly, none to do with Mille. It is mostly the boy in the bed next to us. I am not aware of his condition, though he is clearly neurologically unwell and spends the night throwing his possessions out of bed with some force. I'd guess he must be about twelve. What's puzzling is that rather than providing soft toys for him to toss about, his mother gives him plastic pots and jars of various descriptions. As he noisily throws them out, she puts them back on his bed for him to repeat this meaningless task – the absurdity of the myth of Sisyphus finally explained in the most unusual of circumstances. It's amazing what a day and a half of living with a daughter with cancer does to your tolerance level. I turn away and go back to sleep.

As I drift into somnolence, I am acutely aware of the little foresight I am afforded in the current situation. This becomes a recurring theme. I know nothing of what the future holds for me, for my family, for Millie. My head is firmly reversed and set the contrary to the rest of my body. I can only see the events as they have unfolded. I am also keenly aware of the resolve growing within me, the steadfast determination that is taking over my body and driving me to tirelessly dedicate myself and my time to making Millie better over the coming months; and of course, a newly gained and emergent sense of perspective.

The darkness that surrounds me does not scare me any longer. My duty, my obligation, my responsibility is to commit here and now to Millie and her recovery, for as long as it takes. I made her. It was my choice to bring her into the world, not hers – therefore she owes me nothing and I owe her everything. No questions asked. I fall into a deep and peaceful sleep.

The nurse (a bloke) looking after Millie this first night has been amazing. Millie has had a good night overall. Her 'obs' (observations) have been steady (they have been taken every hour – blood pressure, heart rate, blood count etc.) and the urine output shows clear indications of a diagnosis of diabetes insipidus. I can't help but feel that this should have been made a year ago by any endocrinologist worth his name, though clearly not the one we went to see, despite being of good repute. Or I might just be suffering from hindsight bias.

Vanessa soon joins me. Millie wakes from time to time. She responds well to questions but is clearly visually impaired, and has the empty gaze of the blind. She hears our voices, but cannot make eye contact. She is drinking but not eating much. Vanessa takes her turn to stay with Millie and I go for a nap in the single room, where I fall asleep instantly until about 8am.

We begin to get accustomed to ward routine – a team of doctors do the rounds in the morning, then various specialists begin to come and see us. We are only at the beginning of a long process, but in the next few days we will connect with consultants covering:

- Neurosurgery (brain surgeon)
- Oncology (yes, we'll discover later it's cancer)
- Nephrology (kidney doctor; renal function is closely monitored when undergoing chemotherapy, as Millie will later in the month. Yippee!)
- Endocrinology (hormone doctor)
- Physiotherapy (to establish if motor-neuron skills have been affected, and to what degree she can navigate the

world around her now that she is blind and now that she has undergone major brain surgery)

- Ophthalmology (eye doctor – it is an unfortunate paradox that the eye doctors will often prove to be the most difficult to see at GOSH)
- Audiology (ear doctor – one of the side effects of undergoing chemotherapy is possible hearing loss. Gradual disclosure again, my good loyal friend…)

That's more 'ologies' than you can shake a stethoscope at, and I'm sure I'm missing a few. Over the coming weeks I learn much of each of those specialisms, and some extra ones just for kicks. I will learn to admire some and loathe others.

The day is quite disjointed and all a bit of a blur. I am aware Margaret Thatcher is constantly on the television by the ward's reception, where I go and make coffee. I guess she must have died. I briefly reflect on how lucky she was to live to eighty-seven and to have had the opportunity to achieve so much (some would disagree…), compared to poor Millie May, who may struggle to finish school, if she gets to finish at all.

Millie is in a state of semi-sleep for much of the day. She is not eating, but still asks for water regularly. Endocrine begin their work on Millie. We meet Prof E for the first time and we like him instantly (unlike the multitude of endocrine staff and registrars who will make our life and that of Millie's quite unpleasant over the coming weeks, though admittedly through no fault of their own). He immediately confirms the diagnosis of diabetes insipidus (not to be confused with the much more common type of diabetes, diabetes mellitus. The two conditions are not related). Finally, some closure on a problem we have had for the last year. It is odd to experience relief about the diagnosis of a relatively bothersome disorder.

53

Diabetes insipidus is a condition in which the ability to control the balance of water within the body does not work properly. The kidneys are not able to regulate water balance and retention, and this means that large amounts of dilute urine are passed. Because of this, the body compensates with increased thirst and a lot more drinking. Up to twenty litres of water a day for some, though Millie only manages up to about six – or a third of her body weight. You also enter a world where the words 'sodium' and 'potassium' are mentioned with painful regularity. I have yet to have a conversation – and I've had many – with an endocrine doctor where the word sodium isn't mentioned at least once.

While in hospital, Millie's sodium levels need to be checked three times a day before taking a medicine to counteract her thirst. This means taking her blood three times a day, and when she's not hooked up to an arterial line, as she is at the moment, or some other device which will later be used for chemotherapy (Hickman line – more on that later), it means pricking her fingers or injections every time. This will be the case in the coming days, though gradual disclosure means we don't know it yet.

There are two different types of diabetes insipidus and Millie has cranial diabetes insipidus. Her tumour probably damaged some of the cells in the pituitary responsible for releasing a hormone called ADH (antidiuretic hormone). ADH helps the kidneys to concentrate urine. If less ADH is released, an increased volume of dilute urine is passed, as has been the case for Millie. They are still trying to get the dose right (we are talking micrograms here, so minute) but even ten micrograms of a drug called desmopressin, three times a day, has an immediate effect. The thirst stops as if by magic. The downside is that she will need to take it three times a day *for the rest of her life*.

Having elderly parents, I am familiar with regular drug taking, but some mental adjustment is required to think that *ad infinitum* drug taking will also apply to my seven-year-old daughter. Desmopressin won't be the only drug either. Millie will also be on some sort of steroid three times a day and a medicine to prevent ulcers and tummy upsets caused by intake of steroid. A medicine to counteract the nasty side effects of a medicine that is taken to make you better is a good commercial model if nothing else – especially if you happen to manufacture both drugs.

So here's how I adjust my mental state. I tell myself we all suffer from certain restrictions in life. I need to wear glasses from the moment I wake up in the morning, or else I can't drive my car, watch television or do computer work. Even without going into mild disabilities, we all, as human beings, need to eat and drink a certain amount of food and water every day, otherwise we quite simply die. It is a massive restriction, but we don't think anything of it, simply because it forms part of the natural state of affairs of being human. If you are in an environment with no food or water, you're given a sharp reminder of this restriction, especially when there is proximity between, say, not drinking and suffering severe dehydration – in the desert for example. Indeed, our attitude to water is very different in that environment, much like our attitude to medicine-taking when it, too, becomes essential. Taking a pill with your three main meals every day is simply no big deal when you consider the alternative, which is the same one as not eating or drinking. Millie is seven, and by the time she is eight (if she gets there – at this stage in the proceedings, we just don't know), regular pill-taking will just become part of her routine. Like eating breakfast, brushing her teeth or flossing.

As often happens when faced with events outside of one's control, I try and build justifications, I normalise, I put a spin on the situation and skew my interpretation of reality. Anything to help me cope with the inescapable fact that my daughter has a brain tumour still growing inside her head (and which we will discover tomorrow morning is actually malignant cancer), is blind and will require hormone replacement for the rest of her life.

We manage a second night as a duo, Vanessa and me, but from tomorrow, we'll need to start thinking about just one of us staying and the other going to the flat in the evening. It is the least of our problems, as we are soon reminded.

# THERE IN THE DEPTH WE
# SAW A PAINTED TRIBE

*22) Day 5 – 9:49am, Tuesday 9th April 2013*

Or the day we find out Millie has a rare malignant cancer of the brain.

Last night was similar to the first, though Vanessa stayed with Millie this time. We understand the need to preserve our energies and so begin to approach this as a tag team of two, for the time being. Given Millie's current state, it's really just a matter of being close to her in case she gains a few minutes of consciousness. Her eyes are now swollen and she is unable to open them, so we can't really make an assessment on whether or not she can see. The one glimmer of hope is that both pupils are reactive to light (the good eye on the left more so than the other). And that means at least some light is going through; how much light we still don't know. An ophthalmologist came up but couldn't make a proper assessment given the swelling.

We meet Millie's oncologist for the first time. I'm familiar with the term. Unfortunately. Fortunately, Dr H is a delightful chap – I have to stop liking consultants on first impressions. He tells us that following a review of her tumour marker results from recent blood samples, Millie's tumour is not, in fact, an astrocytoma (or, as originally thought, a craniopharyngioma). It is actually a very rare form of cancer called a secreting germ cell tumour. Ah yes, and it's malignant. About ten children a year in the UK are diagnosed with it (rotten luck on an astronomical scale) and so it changes the plan somewhat with regards to how it will be treated. By this stage, after four days of emotional battering, we have been kicked so hard and for so long that we are on the floor unconscious. The meanies can keep on kicking us, but we just don't feel a thing (the bruises when we wake up will hurt, however). We are unmoved by this latest piece of news, even though we should be devastated. The plan is this:

- As we are dealing with cancer, there will definitely be chemotherapy. Protocol suggests that the most effective treatment is four cycles of chemotherapy over the next three to four months. The first cycle will probably start at the end of next week.
- It is likely that Millie will need a second brain operation following these four courses of chemotherapy (actually, that will happen soon after the second course) to remove whatever is left inside. Some elements of the lump are benign, so chemo does not deal with them.
- Radiotherapy will follow, starting when Millie would have been due to begin her fifth session of chemotherapy.

Dr H tells us that the prognosis associated with this type of cancer has been much improved by the use of what the medical profession call 'multimodality of treatment' (i.e. surgery, chemo and radiotherapy), though I begin to doubt what, if any, quality of life Millie will have if she is 'cured' of cancer. Over 65%

progression-free survival is reported in children. But that means 35% do not survive, so cancer kills one in three – let's hope it's not Millie. Even with my vague understanding of statistics, I presume that there is probably a margin of error in that 65%. Besides, with just ten children suffering secreting germ cell tumour a year in the UK, God knows how they arrive at statistically meaningful figures (maybe they consult worldwide?). As far as I am concerned, malignant cells will either react to chemotherapy at the level of the individual or they won't. So that's 100% successful or 0% successful as far as Millie is concerned. This makes it more like 50:50 and less like 65%.

In the depth of Millie's brain, the painted tribe turned out to be mobs of malignant cancerous cells, which may well end up taking her life. I stop thinking for a while.


*23) Day 5 – 1:09pm, Tuesday 9th April 2013*

I have been significantly more regular from a toilet perspective since the diagnosis. Not that I needed to. I was regular before, but over the last five days, I've been going three times a day on average. I haven't been home to weigh myself yet, but when I do in two days' time, I'll find out that I have lost nearly a stone in seven days. At sixty-eight kilos and 1.82m, I wasn't exactly large to begin with, but the stress is clearly taking its toll (not a diet I would recommend to anyone…). We had been forewarned to make sure that in looking after Millie, we didn't forget to also look after ourselves (Vanessa lost a good four kilos too) but I wasn't quite expecting this event to have such a dramatic impact on my weight.

Millie, meanwhile, is still not eating, but she is on fluid replacement and the doctors don't seem overly concerned. Poor little thing. My mind keeps going back to when she was well, and I keep wondering what will become of us, of her. Silence and solitude bring darkness to my thoughts, but I mustn't lose myself in them. I have to keep focusing on the task ahead. And I refuse to feel sorry for Millie. That would be doing Millie a huge disservice. Vanessa and I will carry on making sure she is the best she can be, but we know it's going to be hard. We know it will take a long time of big ups and massive downs – of unexpected turns on the road, of curve balls and acts of God (I don't mean that in a religious sense).

News of Millie's condition is starting to trickle down to our local community; mums from school, that sort of thing. Some messages of goodwill are beginning to filter through and a lot of them contain religious themes or the vocabulary of warfare. Neither is my cup of tea. I have never been a religious person. We didn't go to church when I was young. Both my parents were scientists, and whilst both were brought up in a Christian environment, neither were/are particularly religious. If there was an omnipotent God, capable of miracle cancer cures, I would find it an odd paradox that he would allow Millie to get cancer in the first place to then have to spend time and energy redressing that. Unless, of course, he suffered from incorrigible narcissism or hero syndrome maybe, and struck down the innocents only to lend them a helping hand to get back up.

If there *is* a God, he is *de facto* responsible for Millie's condition, and I won't write here what I think of such a God. And if there is a God capable of healing Millie, why stop there? Why not cure cancer altogether? I am aware of the easy defence of this from religious corners to say that while God created all, he has no longer any control over it. But that's a non-explanation as far as I'm concerned, as are much of the delusional doctrines, ultimately grounded on wish-thinking, surrounding all religions, from the beginning of time. In any case, God won't help Millie, but orthodox medicine might. I'll side with the latter.

I am still able to accept people's good wishes, however, even if they are dressed in religious cloth. I appreciate the kindness and support they want to express through a medium that provides them with comfort – and if that's Jesus, Allah or Buddha, then so be it.

My other pet hate, as it turns out, is the language of war when it comes to cancer. As if somehow accepting the disease with greater stoicism than the next person will somehow modify the DNA in your cancerous cells to be more receptive to chemotherapy. It may be appealing when it applies to an adult and the treatment of cancer happens to be successful, but significantly less so when it isn't. As if *losing* the *battle* against cancer was somehow a direct cause of not being brave enough, or tenacious enough, or somehow being a lesser person altogether than the person for whom treatment did work, or who had a type of cancer that responded more positively to radiotherapy. What about when we are talking of a seven-year-old girl who can barely spell *brave* or *courageous*? Should they be rid of cancer only if they are worthy warriors? Millie has no concept of what is happening to her, no understanding of the more sinister connotations of her condition. Should I inform her of those lest she doesn't fight arduously enough? Of course not! Nonsense on an astronomical scale.

Talking about messages of goodwill, I really ought to inform Millie's school that she won't be starting the summer term. So I drop an email for the attention of the headmaster (it also happens to be Ellie and Luca's school). Everyone is still on holiday but at least I've set the ball rolling.

In fact, I really ought to formally let all my friends know about Millie. It seems the right thing to do, and also writing about it helps me to distance myself emotionally from the day-to-day gruelling reality of having just discovered Millie has malignant cancer of the brain. It's my cure, so to speak. Not unlike this diary, in a sense. I am jotting down thoughts and significant events of the day on my iPad in order to preserve the vividness of what has unfolded over the past few days. Externalising my angst in this way helps me deal with the situation. I'll take anything at this stage – even writing! It is unexpected. I have never liked writing much.

Something else unexpected happens. Vanessa and I close ranks. We feel an irresistible need to stick together and I discover that love is a *reflex* in these tragic circumstances. Vanessa and I have had a few arguments over the years, as any normal couples do; perhaps more so of late as a result of my own nervy outlook on turning forty last year, of ten years of marriage, of the responsibility felt in having to raise three young children, and of the amount of money that seems to leave our household every month. Call it perspective, a sudden changed outlook on life, or a natural pre-disposition to rely on your loved ones in times of crisis, the fact remains: we start loving each other more (let's hope it's a passing phase!).

Millie is stable and still on morphine. She seems peaceful, pain-free and unburdened by the heaviness that fills our own hearts at fathoming the multitude of tasks and hurdles that lie ahead, at the suffering she will endure and at how much worse she will be before she gets better.

But I'm not in the mood for predicting calamities. I'm not in the mood for self-pity, come to that. *One shot at a time*, I remind myself. One shot at a time.

# FOR AS TIME WEARS ME, I
# SHALL GRIEVE THE MORE

*25) Day 6 – 11:32am, Wednesday 10th April*

The medical profession needs to manage a fine balance between telling the truth – the ugly, unbiased, objective truth – and not sounding unnecessarily alarmist. I understand the concept of managing expectations. Before operation: "Be prepared for all these awful things happening to Millie, they are a real possibility." After operation: "It went very well, I'm very pleased." Gradual disclosure is less of a managed process and more of a necessity, in many ways. When dealing with the body, and in particular something as complex as curing a little girl of cancer, unforeseen events do occur, and they tend to shift the ever-moving goalposts. Treatment needs to adapt. At the same time, I wish the doctors had been more forthcoming about some of the tests Millie would have to undertake to manage the risks associated with *curing* cancer. In other words, she may well get worse as a result of the aggressive therapy required to get rid of her secreting germ cell tumour (or 'latent side effects' as they are often called).

Here are some of the tests and procedures that will be needed while in the neurosurgical ward. There will be more gradual disclosure tests when we move to the chemo ward:

- Millie will undergo another operation in the next couple of days in order to insert a Hickman line. This is a central venous catheter used for the administration of chemotherapy as well as for the withdrawal of blood for analysis (the latter will prove so useful in Millie's case). The insertion of a Hickman line involves two incisions, one at the jugular vein (at the base of the neck) and one in the chest wall. The latter being where the lumens (little white tubes) can be seen coming out. The catheter is advanced into the superior vena cava, near the junction with the right atrium of the heart (what?!). Where the lumen enters the skin it is held down by a stitch and a sterile gauze, which also prevents potential contamination. Potential complications arising from the placement of such a line include haemorrhage and pneumothorax (abnormal collection of air or gas in the space that separates the lung from the chest wall – the pleural space) during insertion and thrombosis or infection at later stages. Patients with a Hickman line require regular flushes of the catheter in order to prevent the line becoming blocked by blood clots. Preventing contamination at the exit site is especially important for oncology patients, as they often become immuno-compromised (medical euphemism for *zero* immunity against bacteria and viral infections) as a result of cytotoxic chemotherapy (an oxymoron).
- CSF analysis (cerebral spinal fluid). This involves a lumbar puncture (a similar procedure to an epidural) to confirm whether or not the cancer has spread beyond the primary site, which, we are told, is a possibility (gradual disclosure!). Luckily, this can be done at the same time as the Hickman line under general anaesthetic.
- A kidney scan and kidney function test (or GFR:

glomerular filtration rate). This measures the flow of filtered fluid by injecting a dye and measuring blood at certain intervals to establish rate of filtration by the kidneys. Chemotherapy is aggressively cytotoxic (i.e. venomous at the cellular level – there's no other word for it), so the kidneys, as natural filters of the body, often take a battering. It is important to ascertain their continuous efficiency and function (critical during chemotherapy), so a test is done prior and several during to compare battered kidney against healthy kidney.

So that's three tests measuring potentially serious implications we didn't know about until this morning.


26) *Day 6 – 1:59pm, Wednesday 10th April*

The nurses confirm to us that Millie is now well enough to be moved from the high dependency ward to a room by herself (and us with her). That's good news, and she is beginning to show signs of life beyond the odd moment awake. She has started listening to music on her iTouch (favourite song: 'From Here to the Moon and Back' by Dolly Parton). Her eyes are still swollen and she sings the words in her darkness. I don't know what she is thinking but we try and talk to her all the time. We tell her she will get better, that feeling rotten after such a big operation is normal, that the swelling in her eyes will go down, that she will be able to open them again before long, and that soon all of this will be behind us.

How do you tell a seven-year-old she may never see again? Her eyes do react to light, so there is hope, but it's all so slow. She can make out a few things with one eye, but not the other.

She still has great difficulty in grabbing the beaker of water that we hand her from time to time. If we keep something very close and very still, five times out of ten, she gets close to guessing what it might be.

A couple of her lines also come out. The arterial line comes out. This is bad. Because she's not hooked up with a Hickman line yet, it means the blood tests she requires three times a day need to be performed the old-fashioned way – needle or prick test, adding to the discomfort she is already under. The head drain comes out too. This is good and relatively painless. I think she has eaten half a piece of one popcorn flake so far and vomited shortly thereafter, but little by little her appetite returns and she starts interacting a little more with the outside world. Millie has now been bedridden for nearly three days, and although it doesn't sound like much, the physiotherapist seems to think it is time we try to get her sitting on the bed, and perhaps attempt to take a few steps. I guess we need to encourage the firing of all neurons, including those that are used for walking around, to help her long-term recovery.

It's difficult to get Millie up. The cumulative effect of the eight-hour brain operation, morphine, diabetes insipidus and the steroid they have started giving her as a precaution is taking its toll (she might need cortisol replacement – also known as the stress hormone because the body secretes more of it during times of stress, both physical and emotional). After ten minutes of motivating her to sit up, she finally acquiesces to give it a try, I think more to be left alone afterwards, than anything else. She does so for about three seconds, is unwilling to stand, but we take that as a small achievement. The physiotherapist also checks Millie's motor skills by getting her to push hard on her hand with both feet, to squeeze with both her hands and move each leg in a certain way.

The physiotherapist then suggests organising a wheelchair for when Millie is discharged. A wheelchair! For my daughter? What are they on about? Surely she won't need a wheelchair? The unfortunate truth is that she might. Fortunately, luck would be on our side for once, and Millie would regain full motor skills after recovering from this brain operation, and indeed the next one (oh, and the one after that…).

Millie's maternal grandmother, Mama, comes to visit and Millie smiles for the first time in three days. I take the opportunity to go and freshen up at the flat and meet my co-directors for coffee. I recount the events of the past few days, and find comfort in seeing them both and being able to think about something other than GOSH, Millie or her tumour. As finance director of the business, all I really need is a laptop and an internet connection, so although they don't expect it, I reassure them I will be able to cover the minimum necessary to fulfil my obligations to the company. The message from them is one of unequivocal support. I am very grateful.

I also let my closest friend Mark know – the only one I have been able to break the bad news to. We were each other's best man, though I did a significantly lesser job of it at his wedding than he did at mine. (Sorry Mark. Here's me apologising. Again.) His words of support help tremendously, and he would help in many other ways over the coming months. He was my only friend who took the time to come and visit me and Millie whilst in hospital, and on several occasions. It won't be forgotten.

I am conscious I ought to let all my other friends know too, so I start drafting an email and recounting recent events. I become acutely aware of the darkness that has engulfed me as a result of what's been happening. I have tried so hard not to show it over the last few days, staying focused for Millie and my family, that the sadness in my heart has crept up unnoticed, like a thief in the night, and stolen much of the sunshine away.

The only light remaining is that of numberless flames exposing the depth of dejection in the very core of my soul.


## 27) Day 6 – 5:41pm, Wednesday 10th April

One such painful flame is further fanned by certain mid-level endocrinologists back at GOSH, who confirm that Millie's operation to 'install' her Hickman line is now scheduled for Friday. This is the intravenous tube that will be used to poison her body with cytotoxic drugs during chemotherapy. Now that her arterial line has been taken out, endocrinology needs to measure her sodium level before each dose of desmopressin, by taking blood with finger pricks or by accessing a vein with a needle. Millie is upset and it seems an unnecessary torture, especially after all that has happened.

For the first time since being admitted at GOSH I feel helpless. After four days of intensive effort, I realise Millie has now been integrated into the administrative workings of an NHS hospital; an excellent one, but not perfect by any means. In particular, it seems prone to the same deficiencies of many of the large corporations I have worked for over the last twenty years. Sometimes, the drive to follow process overrides common sense and stifles the ability of mid-level doctors to think for themselves. Doing the right thing for the client (Millie) becomes a process of ticking boxes in accordance with whatever condition is being treated at the time. In the context of endocrine, that means taking blood before administering every dose of desmopressin three times a day. This is despite the fact Millie has managed to balance her fluid with the condition for the last year, that her sodium has been fine for the last two days, and that soon they would send us home and we would give her the drug three times a day without stabbing a needle in her vein every time. So at home there's no risk, but as soon as you enter the confines of an NHS hospital, risk crystallises? It's not the first time I have a run-in with endocrine for trying to implement a process that is counter-productive to what they are trying to achieve. More on this later. Endocrine, I'm not finished with you yet.

After some kicking and screaming, Millie finally agrees to let us prick her finger. Her sodium levels are normal. She can be given the drug – wouldn't you know it! A drug, by the way, which at the dose currently given to Millie, has the same level of risk attached to it as eating a spoonful of porridge.

# SO WERE MINE EYES
# INEBRIATE THAT THEY
# LONGED TO STAY AND WEEP

*28) Day 7 – Thursday 11th April*

It's all relative of course, but the intensity of the last six days is slowly declining. From a frame of reference that did not allow us to look beyond the next few hours, our outlook can now extend to a full twenty-four-hour period. Progress? Or perhaps we're learning how to cope better. I feel like I have aged sixty years in six days.

Part of the learning process, and perhaps my own emotional cure, has been to write. I keep notes of the day, of how I feel about it all. I also feel the need to share the news with my friends. I think they deserve to know, not least to avoid any awkward conversations when I next see some of them. I need to equip them with the knowledge that will enable them to say the right thing when we meet. Partly also, the urge to share is possibly a narcissistic attempt at finding comfort from the knowledge that others share in my grief, that I am loved, and that I'm not alone.

I write them all an email.

*Dear all*

Apologies for the round-robin general email. I felt it was right to update you, as friends, old and new, on recent events. Please respect the private nature of this email by not forwarding it on to anyone else.

It is with immense sadness that I write to let you know that our seven-year-old daughter Millie May has been diagnosed with a secreting germ cell tumour (malignant brain cancer that occurs in no more than ten children a year in the UK. Rotten luck on an astronomical scale).

It all happened very quickly, and I am writing this email during a quiet moment at Great Ormond Street Hospital, where Vanessa and I are spending much of our time during this early phase.

On Friday 5th April, we were due to go to London to take Millie to see our paediatrician as she was complaining of feeling a little poorly. Nothing too unusual. As we were leaving for London it became apparent that she had sudden loss of vision in her right eye and limited vision in her left. An hour later, up in London, she was rushed for an MRI scan, which confirmed that she had a brain tumour, probably originating close to the pituitary gland (so, deep within the brain). Our paediatrician managed to get us into GOSH and meet the neurosurgical team at 10am on the Saturday. Following other tests, and in order to try and preserve the little eye sight she had left, she was admitted into theatre on Sunday morning for brain surgery, in an attempt to remove a sufficient amount of tumour to release pressure on the optic nerve (the cause of the vision loss).

The surgery took approximately eight hours, and we are now in the process of planning for the many difficult stages that will follow. After four days of gradual disclosure by various

*medical teams, many turns in the road and many uncertainties,*
*we now know roughly where we might possibly be ('roughly',*
*'might' and 'possibly' being the operative words):*

- *We are still unclear to what degree, if at all, Millie has regained her sight.*
- *She will begin chemotherapy in a couple of weeks, for four months, following another minor operation to put in a line to allow unintrusive access for the chemical mix and various blood tests she will require over the next four months.*
- *This particular type of cancer responds well to chemotherapy and radiotherapy, and there is a 65% chance of success, though the road ahead is considerably more complex, winding and tortuous then the simplistic statistic suggests.*

*We have had the good fortune of 100% support from our family. It has allowed Vanessa and me to concentrate entirely on Millie over the last four days.*

*Hope is a currency we cannot allow ourselves to use at this stage, but Vanessa and I are determined to be the best we can be for Millie. Our resolve and focus to hold her hand through this difficult journey is steadfast.*

*Much love to all*
*Marco and Vanessa*

Reading back the email as part of the process of writing this book a few months down the line, some of the darkness has dissipated. Or perhaps experience plays a part in easing the pain. Experience is a cruel teacher, but we certainly learn. Hope is still a currency we can seldom use, but some of the events that will unfold in the next few months will restore some optimism, though we know we need to keep it in check for much of the time. There are too many ups and downs along the way to allow our emotions to feel anything other than steady numbness. It's a survival mechanism, and we need to be that way for Millie's sake. Our determination to be the best we can be has only grown.

Mrs Thatcher is still in the news and they show some clips of her time in office, including the one where she speaks in the aftermath of the Brighton hotel bombing. She begins the conference at 9:30am the following day as an act of defiance: "The fact that we are gathered here now, shocked but composed and determined." Shocked. Composed. Determined. It's how Vanessa and I feel. We refuse to even think of diminishing the level of effort we know is required in the long term to make Millie better. It's not about us, it's about Millie.


## 29) Day 8 – Friday 12th April: am

The darkness I speak of in my email makes it difficult to see as we continue our descent into the dread abyss. This morning, Millie will have an operation to have her Hickman line put in; one step closer to chemotherapy, which nothing can truly prepare you for. We have a meeting with Millie's oncologist, Dr H, and he gives us a broad outline about what to expect, together with a few leaflets explaining the course of treatment Millie will be subjected to.

She is likely to follow PEI protocol. It's pronounced 'pie', like the one you eat and so called because it's an abbreviation of the delightful substances which are injected directly in the blood stream: cisplatin (the P of PEI – go figure), etoposide and ifosfamide. More on these lovely liquids in the next section. She will have four courses of chemotherapy over four months (so one week of treatment, three weeks off, one week of treatment, three weeks off etc.). The weeks off are there to allow the body to recover. These strong drugs are cytotoxic, killing fast-growing cancer cells in the body but also other fast-growing cells like white blood cells and those that produce hair. This accounts for the hair loss normally associated with patients undergoing chemotherapy, and their general lack of immunity during treatment.

Another of the drug's side effects, Dr H tells us, is the possible deterioration of Millie's hearing. I'm not sure whether this is because hair cells in the ear allow us to hear by sending electrical impulses that are then translated into sound by the brain. Analogue data turned into digital data every time you hear a sound – amazing. As she's nearly blind, Dr H is keen to avoid deafness too (as are we!), so wants to monitor it closely. We are going to have a hearing test to establish Millie's baseline, and then keep on testing it as chemotherapy progresses.

So we're in it for the next four months, after which Millie may or may not require a further brain operation to remove what remains – if there's still some tumour left. She may or may not be blind, and now, as it turns out, may or may not be deaf. We have been doing this for six days now and four months is a time frame I find difficult to process.

The operation goes well, and Millie has an MRI scan and lumbar puncture at the same time to check fluid and see if the cancer has spread. She also now has a lumen sticking out of her flank. It's not pleasant to see your daughter with a tube inserted into the side of her chest, going all the way into her body, through which a toxic cocktail of medicine will do damage beyond our current understanding.

Meanwhile, Millie is gaining her appetite post-op and asks

to be taken on a little outing in one of the ward's wheelchairs. As I walk around with her, I discreetly try and ask her about what she sees. Koala Ward has koalas and other jungle animals painted on the walls. She can make out the Koalas, but only when she is very close, and certainly cannot see big writing of any description, even the two-foot-tall floor numbers above the lifts, or the large fire exit signs. Nevertheless, we feel there is some improvement in her eyes and this is confirmed by ophthalmology later today.

Tests show that with her good eye, she can see large pictures (A4 size) at two meters away when they are not moving. It's something! There's nothing still from the other eye, though both are still reactive to light. The eye doctor also confirms that we should know for sure about potential improvement when she has an electro-retinogram. During this process electrodes are placed on your head, light is shone into your eyes, and the electrodes record brain activity, thus measuring the amount of light that goes through the optic nerve, like cable bandwidth. The eye doctor also says that there is very little that can be done, as the physiology of the eye is as it should be. What's 'broken' is the optic nerve – and, as with all nerve cells, once they're dead, they're dead. So glasses won't help, nor will any operations. If that's all she can see, that's all she can see. How's that for hope value? We are also told that every patient is different so it is difficult to make predictions about possible improvement (a standard reply in hospitals). Some tell us improvements are normally seen in the first three to four weeks, others mention up to six months, and others still suggest that even after a couple of years, improvements (if they happen, that is) do materialise.

I am finding this vision thing worrying. It's getting to me a little bit. But we've got it good at the moment, as I find out when Millie starts chemotherapy a week or so from now. Her start date has not yet been confirmed and we are having to do some chasing. In fact, we are learning that things happen more quickly if you get personally involved in following up outstanding activities. So we start politely reminding nurses, head nurses and doctors at every opportunity about who we want to see, what tests are outstanding, what confirmation we await and from which department. Chasing for things to happen will also become a feature of our future stays in hospital.


## 30) Day 8 – Friday 12th April: pm

I call Ellie Rose, my nine-year-old daughter. I'm mindful I haven't spoken or seen her for six days now and although she is staying with her aunty and Mama, who she loves, I want to make sure she knows she's still loved and remembered as the focus begins to shift from her and Luca to be redirected almost entirely towards Millie May, for the next three to four months at least. She knows Millie is unwell and that she's had an operation, but nothing beyond that. I know I will have to explain to her, in a language she can understand, what Millie and we as a family are going through. I don't want to do it over the phone, however, nor do I want to deceive her under false pretences. I need to do it face to face. I need to see her reaction and gauge my vocabulary accordingly.

I find it difficult not to cry as I hear her voice and tell her that I love her and miss her very much. She seems happy – that's all that matters.

# TURNING OUR BACK UPON
# THE VALE OF WOE

*31) Day 9 – Saturday 13th April*

Millie's catheter is coming out this morning – the last tube to come out from when she had brain surgery. The catheter stays in place because of a little balloon of water placed in the bladder itself. Removing it is simple. There is a small access lock at the base of the catheter and you simply lock in a syringe, extract the water (so deflate the balloon) and gently pull the device out. What they don't tell you are the complications that can result from having a catheter removed, including being unable to release urine and the need to reinsert one without the benefit of general anaesthetic. Luckily this does not happen to Millie, but it does mean that from now on, because her input and output (drink and wee) are still being measured, she has to pass urine into a disposal pot that is weighed every time. She seems to take relatively well to this particular intrusion of her privacy. And she can tell whether or not the pot is on the loo seat (so she can see something). So that's good.

We finally get confirmation about the first chemotherapy session. Millie will start next Tuesday and we will be admitted to Elephant Ward for this (start noticing an animal theme? It doesn't make these places any cuter). The ward is up one floor and Millie will be moved later today. Meanwhile, the enormity of the task ahead, and the multiplicity of task management that is going to be required is beginning to play on our minds. How will we juggle chemotherapy, four times in four months as an inpatient for at least five days (Millie actually ends up staying ten days for her first two courses because of complications), my other two childen starting school in a few days, my work etc.? I decide to put my project management skills to the fore.

Firstly, we are going to have to rely on Vanessa's family for the other two children when they start school. School is a complicated business these days, what with school bags, sport kits, netball gear, swimming kits, gym kit and various pick-up and drop-off times. Whilst *we* are familiar with it, we need to somehow share that knowledge with others who will help out. Jonny, Vanessa's brother, is very IT literate and I discuss with him the possibility of having shared calendars on iPads. So we have one calendar for each child and one calendar for stuff relating to the house (predominantly my whereabouts and Vanessa's whereabouts). I feel it's very important to be open about our timetable and activities to let Vanessa's family know where we are, so they can be better equipped to help, to know where they need to be and when, who to pick up and so on and so forth.

For the first time in nine days I go back home to East Sussex to meet Jonny. He picks me up from the station and we go straight to buy two iPad Minis: one for Vanessa and one for her mother. I have one already. Josie, Vanessa's sister, has one already, and Jonny has one. It's a small investment to make for what will prove to be a very useful tool for managing our activities over the next four months. Being that way inclined, I manage the input into this diarised database to make sure it's accurate and up to date. Before going back to GOSH we stop by the house so that I can have a shower and pick up a few things, including a few picture books for Millie.

For the first time in nine days I go back into Millie's room. I smell her smell. My mind betrays me and goes back to happier days, when we didn't know what she had. The events of the last few days unfold, like a fog dispersing gradually, finally revealing the grim reality of the tragedy that has befallen us. The Millie of nine days ago is dead. It is likely we will have to adjust to living with a new Millie – and that's if we're lucky. Fear comes over me. I feel for Millie and all the challenges she will have to face with the many disabilities she might have. For only the second time in nine days, there, alone and in the shadows of a life that will never be the same again, I sit on her bed and let myself cry all the tears in my body; for the last time.

I gather my things, close the door behind me and go to the station to take the train back to GOSH. Back at the hospital, the grim reality of Elephant Ward is hard to take in. As I walk to Millie's room, I see several children in various stages of decomposition, hooked up to chemo, without hair, white of face and deep sadness in their eyes. It's difficult to think Millie will look like that at some point during treatment, as the toxic agents in the drugs take effect on her body. I see parents, tired and sad, but somehow I don't feel sorry for them, or for myself, for having to go through it. Ours is the easy job, that of holding our children's hands as they get pumped full of poison. They are the ones that have to go through it all.

## 32) Day 10 – Sunday 14th April

It's a slow day as we wait for chemotherapy to start on Tuesday. There are still a few tests to be done, including a hearing test (confirmed for tomorrow) and kidney scan and function test, which we will be doing today. These are to establish a baseline for the ears and kidneys, to compare against future results, as Millie goes through her four cycles of chemo.

As I make myself a coffee, I meet another dad. The gloomy affinity that connects us pushes me to engage him in conversation. He tells me his story. His four-and-a-half-month-old son has cancer (diagnosed during pregnancy) and has just completed his 121st day of chemotherapy. I think he said it was neuroblastoma, which sounds a bit like cancer from outer space. So in the same way Millie will have twenty days of chemotherapy in total (five days for each of her four cycles), this chap's been here pretty much since his son was born.

While the population at GOSH is not representative of the world at large (all parents at GOSH have ill children), it would not be the first time I felt humbled by someone else's tragic experience. In time, and it's an unfortunate absurdity, but a real one nonetheless, the realisation there is always someone much worse off in life would actually make me feel relatively lucky that the *only* thing my daughter had was brain cancer.

## 33) Day 11 – Monday 15th April

Chemotherapy starts tomorrow. Millie is still very weak from her operation but has managed a few outings on her own unaided by a wheelchair. She goes to the toilet by herself, holding on to the side of the bed and feeling her way to the bathroom door. Her vision seems to have improved a touch, though she still sees very little. She certainly can't read normal writing, but can make out big letters and numbers if they are written in black ink and the page does not move in front of her.

Her kidney function and kidneys are normal. The kidney scan involves an ultrasound and Millie doesn't enjoy the cold gel much, but other than that it all goes well. The kidney function test takes longer and broadly consists of injecting a dye into her blood stream and then assessing kidney efficiency by measuring glomerular filtration rate at various intervals (by taking blood through her Hickman line prior to injection of the dye, after three hours and then after one hour). Millie will have a kidney function test before and after each session of chemotherapy, essential given the nature of the treatment and the importance of good functioning kidneys in getting rid of the toxic cocktail of chemicals that is injected daily over a period of five days.

We also manage to have a hearing test. The results are broadly normal, with mild high-frequency hearing loss on both sides (probably genetic and nothing to worry about), but without any functional hearing difficulties. The tests themselves are relatively un-intrusive, and I remember them well from childhood, having had grommets on two separate occasions. Grommets, also called a 'tympanostomy tube' are little tubes inserted into the eardrum to allow air to pass through into the middle ear, and thus release any pressure build-up and help clear excess fluid within. Given that the genetic hearing loss is on the maternal side (my wife suffers from it too – or is that selective to filter out the sound of my voice when I ask her to do things around the house?), they would like to test my wife and mother-in-law for good measure – or perhaps just to rub it in. We get it! Our family does not have perfect ears to make out sounds only dogs can hear. I'll live with that.

One of the hearing tests involves Millie throwing a coloured ball into a basket when she hears a sound through some earphones. She misses the basket a couple of times (not important for the hearing test) but other than that can broadly see the basket and feels confident enough to aim and throw with relative ease. This is encouraging from a vision perspective. She soon gets tired of it all though, and we go back to Elephant Ward for some rest.

Millie has now been in hospital for ten days and ten nights. We are conscious she will need to spend at least another five days here while she undergoes chemotherapy and so we are keen, now that all tests are done, to try and have an outing somewhere local as a teatime treat for Millie. We go to Pizza Express and she has her favourite. I never imagined I would enjoy going to that place so much, but the elation is of a kind only enjoyed following a spell in the harshest, most hostile situation I have encountered in my life so far. I know it isn't joy at all. But I take it in nonetheless. I need to feel normal again, if only for a few minutes, to try and regain some proximity to life before cancer, after the last days spent crossing this dark valley filled with grief.

As we return to GOSH, we know this is the first test in the most Herculean of labours to be undertaken over the next few months. We hope we're up to the task. We hope we can be good parents. We hope Millie will pull through without too much damage. We hope she won't suffer during her treatment, or as a result of the cure required to make her better. We hope we will be able to preserve her soul, what makes her Millie, and not just be left with a live body upon this earth. We hope, beyond the realms of what is permissible to hope as a result of her condition. We hope...

# THE WAY IS LONG, AND
# MUCH UNCOUTH THE ROAD

*34) Epilogue to Inferno*

When I had journeyed half of my life's way, I found myself within a shadowed forest. The events that have unfolded over the last eleven days have been the most traumatic, upsetting and hurtful in my life, in Vanessa's life, and in much of our immediate families' lives combined. We were very much caught in a violent storm, unable to stop the sequence of reactions triggered by Millie's loss of vision on that ill-fated Friday morning.

During this brief period of time, my seven-year-old daughter has been diagnosed with a malignant brain tumour (of the rarest kind, and one which could end her life, if not now then possibly in the next few months or years). She may well remain so visually impaired as to qualify as blind, will have to take drugs for the rest of her life to manage a condition that makes her drink litres of water over twenty-four hours, and is likely to require help growing, with daily injections of growth hormones.

Millie still has a lump in her brain, the size of a golf ball, which we now know is a malignant brain tumour, set so deep in her head that any attempt to remove it may well cause further long-term damage that would significantly worsen her quality of life. She will undergo four months of gruelling chemotherapy, and then two months of radiotherapy, which may aggravate the conditions she is currently suffering by further damaging her pituitary gland and hypothalamus. It is likely she will, after chemotherapy and prior to radiotherapy, undergo a second eight-hour brain operation to remove what is left of the tumour; such an operation not being without its material risks (loss of life, total blindness, further worsening of conditions relating to damaging the pituitary gland or hypothalamus).

Perhaps the three most overwhelming themes of the last eleven days have been ones of uncertainty, fear and grief. Uncertainty as to her condition, whether this was the right course of action, what the future will hold in terms of treatment and its success, and to what degree we will be able to cope. Fear about the more sinister and serious nature of her situation. Cancer kills. And Millie has it. Fear of the unknown, of the risks associated with *curing* cancer, especially when it is in a region as sensitive as the brain. Also fear of what might become of Millie, of how much she might suffer over the coming months. And finally: grief. It is clear by now that Millie is not suffering from an illness from which she will recover and return to her normal self. The Millie we knew and loved is dead. Another Millie is evolving in her place as the various treatments take their course and their toll. And, in that sense, we have lost our darling daughter and must get used to it. We can only hope that modern medicine will limit the damage made by her tumour and the inevitable harm the cure will bring – and so preserve as much of Millie as possible, for as long as possible.

Grief demands an answer, but sometimes there isn't one. Being here was inevitable. Millie didn't suffer from a broken leg or an accident we could have avoided. Cancer had been creeping ever closer to the surface, unstoppable, unrelenting, and it was only a matter of time before this monster revealed itself from the murky depths. On balance, while we are in an awful situation, we've done everything we can to manage the storm that descended so abruptly and with such brutal force into our lives.

And, perhaps more importantly, while in shock, we feel composed and determined to see this through for Millie's sake. The certainty that we will be able to cope is reassuring. It will be a while before we behold the stars; but for now we must depart from Hell, this evil place that cancer has built around us, around our hearts and souls. Chemotherapy next – this Purgatory may yet bring us closer to the lights of Heaven. Only time will tell.

# II

# PURGATORIO
## *(PURGATORY)*

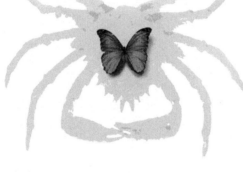

"Per correr miglior acque alza le vele
omai la navicella del mio ingegno,
che lascia dietro a sé mar sì crudele;

e canterò di quel secondo regno
dove l'umano spirito si purga
e di salire al ciel diventa degno."

*"Over better waves to speed her rapid course
The light bark of my genius lifts the sail,
Well pleased to leave so cruel sea behind;*

*And of that second region will I sing,
In which the human spirit from sinful blot
Is purged, and for ascent to Heaven prepares."*

Dante Alighieri, The Divine Comedy
*Purgatorio – Canto I, lines 1-6*

"Millie's mid-chemo course MRI shows that treatment-induced cysts have increased the size of her tumour. We feel the best course of action is to operate as soon as possible. We have a free slot tomorrow morning. Are you able to come up to GOSH this afternoon to be admitted?"
Dr M, oncologist at GOSH covering for Dr H
*19) Day 61 – Tuesday 4th June*

# THAT HUE WHICH THE DUN
# SHADES OF HELL
# CONCEALED

## 1) Day 12 – 10:15am, Tuesday 16th April

It feels good in some way to have "progressed" to chemotherapy; although the road ahead is long and winding. We know it is likely Millie will need another operation to remove whatever chemotherapy cannot kill off. Actually, it ends up being two further operations – but more on that later.

Prior to actually injecting cytotoxic drugs into her system, we go through the usual ceremony of signing for consent – it provides parents with the illusion of control. This time I see Millie's oncologist, Dr H, on my own and he runs through what to expect, both short and long term. One technique for breaking bad news has always been to empower the patient, or in this case the patient's father, to play back their understanding of the situation. It's called 'perception'. It's what Dr H did with us prior to letting us know that what she had was malignant, and it's what he does with me now prior to listing all the lovely things Millie will be afflicted with during treatment. I recall the events of the last eleven days and summarise where I think we are – there is much deliberate acquiescence from Dr H (perception in action).

I have touched on the PEI protocol Millie will follow, but it is perhaps worth another glance. PEI protocol is so called because it's an abbreviation of the 'agents' which are injected directly into the bloodstream: cisplatin (the P of PEI), ifosfamide and etoposide.

Chemotherapy aims primarily to control and reduce the spread of cancer cells in the body. Three primary factors are crucial to the overall success of chemotherapy as a treatment: the specific cocktail of cytotoxic agents used, its quantity, and the timing of when this is given. Cancer chemotherapeutic agents come in various shapes and sizes – broadly ten different categories – and there are about a hundred such drugs that, used in certain combinations, provide the desired effect (sometimes). Cancer treatment through chemotherapy involves the exploitation of the biological characteristics of cancer cells to make them susceptible to drug therapy. In a nutshell – cancer cells are fast-dividing cells, but they are cells nonetheless and so are open to attacks by chemical agents that affect their reproduction. This primarily targets the way in which their DNA replicates, but that's not the only way.

In targeting fast-dividing cancerous cells, chemotherapy also targets other 'healthy' fast-dividing cells. As mentioned before, hair follicles fall into this category – hence the hair loss. Perhaps more significantly, chemotherapy can also affect fertility, another site where fast cell division occurs. I think to myself that, actually, if we are faced with the problem of Millie trying to conceive later in life then I feel we will have been stupendously successful in the context of what she has. The more concerning side effects are immediate, even if relatively minor, because Mille has to deal with them, in particular the more visible ones like hair loss. We'll have to talk to her about that before it actually happens. Another jolly conversation to look forward to.

Back to side effects. Here are other chemotherapy side effects, both temporary and permanent, relating to the specific agents used for Millie's cancer. And these are just the common ones – I'll spare you the occasional or rare ones:

**Temporary side effects:** Hair loss, strange taste, loss of appetite, severe nausea and vomiting, drop in blood pressure, bone marrow suppression, altered kidney function (temporary and possibly permanent), irritation of the bladder wall, disorientation and sleepiness, fluid retention, numbness and tingling, allergic reactions and diarrhoea.

**Permanent side effects:** Hearing loss, altered kidney function (temporary and possibly permanent), second cancer (yes, some chemotherapeutic agents are actually carcinogenic) and fertility (or rather, *in*fertility).

The fight against cancer isn't a fight. It is the careful management of risks against benefits. When dealing with chemical agents so powerful they are able to destroy the very core of cellular structures (i.e. what makes up 100% of you and me), it is no simple matter to implement. Permanent side effects, which often materially and adversely impact quality of life, are an inevitable and paradoxical consequence of *curing* cancer. With the alternative (i.e. not curing cancer), there is no quality of life. This is difficult to stomach, especially when it relates to children, and specifically when it applies to my own seven-year-old daughter, who, until a fortnight ago, was jumping around and playing with my parents' dogs in Italy. Ultimately, the principal goal of chemotherapy (or any therapy, for that matter) is to provide the most beneficial treatment at the lowest risks. 'Most beneficial treatment' and 'risks' are both relative and contextual. There is no black and white in this game of life and death.

I sign the consent form – let's hope the poisonous dew that will be injected directly into my daughter's bloodstream will wash away the cancerous mass that remains, and restore the healthy hue that the grey shades of hell concealed.


## 2) Day 12 – 11:30am, Tuesday 16th April

Most (but not all) chemotherapy causes hair loss – there's no getting away from it. And the one Millie is about to be administered will cause hair loss. As always, we are keen to ensure Millie is kept informed. I know she is only seven, but trust is essential in these extreme circumstances and we have a duty to ensure she knows and understands what is going to happen to her during each phase of treatment. Admittedly, this is an easier conversation than many we've had to dish out over the past two weeks, but hair is such a fundamental and defining feature, especially in a little girl, that we're somewhat apprehensive about letting her know. She has lost so many things in the last fortnight and she is about to lose her dignity. She will now also look different to her peers and friends, and we know it'll knock her confidence.

Feeling normal is an important part of life, and curing cancer often brings with it very visible effects, such as hair loss. This not only makes you feel different – it makes you look different. We know it will upset her and we feel for her. I decide to break the news by telling her that the special medicine that will be injected into her wigglies (Hickman line) is so strong it will not only get rid of the small lump in her head that's making her feel sick – it will also make her hair fall out. The good news, I say, is that her hair will grow back after the treatment is finished in a few months' time. She is, understandably, not very happy with this new information. She asks whether the medicine is absolutely necessary, and is reluctant to take my word for it, so asks to see Dr H.

Very kindly, Dr H agrees to come and be grilled by my seven-year-old, who asks: "Do I have to take these medicines?" "Will they make my hair fall out?" and "Will my hair grow back again after it's finished?" He confirms all three with affirmatives. Millie seems pleased to have been able to have this conversation directly, to somehow feel a little more in control and involved in her ongoing treatment. In our overwhelming desire to protect our sons and daughters, we should never forget that, regardless of their age, they are little people in their own right, with a need to feel empowered to make their own choices, to be involved, and to be treated as individuals with their own independent needs and wants.

The nurses come in to prepare Millie for her first session of chemotherapy – her first of forty-eight intravenous infusions over twenty days, spread across the next four months. The drugs that are being injected will need to be given intravenously over a period of time each day. One drug in particular, cisplatin, is so toxic that Millie will require extra fluid to minimise the risk of kidney damage. This fluid is also given intravenously. Cisplatin is from the family of alkylates as far as chemotherapeutic agents are concerned. It is so called because of the chemical process it causes by effectively breaking down the ability of cells to replicate DNA. Cisplatin works at any point in the cell cycle, and for this reason the effect on the cell is dose dependent; the fraction of cells that die is directly proportional to the dose of the drug. I don't know how much will be injected into Millie's veins, but I do know that this drug is from the family of agents originally derived from mustard gas used in World War I. It will eventually cause acute kidney failure during Millie's second course of chemotherapy in a month's time, and is also the drug that can cause hearing loss – so not your harmless paracetamol.

All in all, fluid of one kind or another will be injected directly into Millie's veins 24/7 for five days. This is at a rate of approximately six to seven litres a day – and that's excluding drinking.

Like a vessel over cytotoxic waves, her body will have to make this journey alone. We can only watch helplessly, like spirits sitting by her side.


*3) Day 12 – 1:45pm, Tuesday 16th April*

Before the chemical onslaught starts, there is time for one more test; and one we have been waiting for anxiously over the past few days: Millie's electro-retinogram test. This will measure how responsive the visual nerve cells are to light.

The tumour, or lesions resulting from it, was putting pressure on the optic nerves. The resulting blood supply deficit was killing off nerve cells, or compressing them (or a combination of both), thus severely affecting Millie's visual fields. In the right eye, the field was reduced to almost nothing, hence the total loss of vision. The left eye got away more lightly – but only just. Millie had lost most of her visual field but retained a small window of light on her nasal side. Defects in the physiology of the eye itself can be rectified (by wearing glasses, for example), but there's little that can be done when nerve cells are compromised. Nerve cells can't be fixed and do not regenerate – when they're dead, they're dead.

The electro-retinogram test was going to tell us the potential for functional improvement in Millie's eyesight. It would measure how much light was going through, how many bits of photons were able to travel through the natural fibre-optic cables of the optic nerves, and to what degree they had been damaged.

I still find the vision impairment aspect of her condition hard to stomach. She can see something, but certainly not enough to get by on her own at the moment. She can see if the door is open or shut when she is standing right in front of it. But she struggles to make out anything that is not still, big or in very close proximity to her face. And no one can tell if she will improve. The objective of the first operation was to preserve the little vision she had left. So far, I think that was achieved but we are still hoping for improvement for her sake.

Different doctors predict different outcomes and paths of progression. "Around 50% of the overall improvement comes in the first three to six weeks." "Improvements are progressive and can happen up to five years after the operation." "After six months, it is unlikely to improve any further." "Improvement begets further improvement, and if no improvement is seen in the first few weeks, it is very unlikely that any progress will be seen thereafter." So, customary for anyone who works in the medical profession, no one commits and no one has a definitive answer. So far, we've noticed a small recovery, but hardly perceptible.

It's one thing living in the aftermath of cancer, with diabetes insipidus and other hormone deficiencies, but with good functional vision. It's another altogether to do so without perceiving any shadows except those cast by your own body.

# WE THROUGH THE BROKEN
# ROCK ASCENDED

*4) Day 12 – 4pm, Tuesday 16th April*

My other two children, Ellie Rose and Luca Jack, have been staying at Vanessa's mother's house for the last twelve days. Summer term starts tomorrow and we've been trying to figure out how we will manage the next three to four months, juggling life, Millie's chemotherapy and school. Vanessa and I have always tried to share responsibility and we know this is no different – we are two able-bodied adults and we are effectively interchangeable as far as looking after Millie or our other two children is concerned.

Ultimately, it is our responsibility to look after *all* of our children, and while the help we have received from Vanessa's family has been invaluable over the course of the last fortnight, we know it is now time to re-establish some form of normality – to relieve Mama and Josie, Vanessa's mother and sister, who have been amazing during the last twelve days, supporting us and looking after Ellie and Luca. We are also aware that the nature of Millie's cure will probably comprise two distinct phases. The intensive phase of treatment, that we are living at the moment, and which will include chemotherapy over the next four months, another two brain operations and then radiotherapy. The second phase, if we get there, is still currently undefined because of the huge number of uncertainties we still have (will chemotherapy be effective? Will a second operation, if she needs one, be successful in removing the lump that chemotherapy has not killed off?) What we do know at this stage is that it is likely to include some form of long-term maintenance or support for the first five years. Though we can barely think beyond the next month, there is a third phase, of course, and that is the ongoing management of Millie's body throughout her lifetime. She will require medication for the rest of her life, that much is clear, and she will need to manage this ongoing maintenance herself as an adult. Our job is to get her there, looking and feeling as normal as we can possibly achieve.

The first intensive phase will require careful organisation and, more importantly, preservation of energy to make sure we can last the distance, for Millie's sake. We can't both be involved all of the time. And we need to gratefully accept help whenever it is offered. So we decide to split our time in hospital 50:50. Vanessa (and often her mother – how can we ever thank her enough) will do two days and two nights, then I will take over and do two days and two nights.

The chemotherapy ward at GOSH is an intense place, both physically and emotionally, where harsh medicine is dished out on a daily basis, with devastating effects on the body. This will be the case when the venomous toxins of cisplatin, ifosfomide and etoposide come into full effect over the course of Millie's treatment. We have both been in hospital for twelve days now, and it's time we implement this job-share arrangement. Vanessa does not feel ready to re-engage with day-to-day school life and, in particular, having to talk about Millie's illness with other mums at school. She finds that aspect particularly difficult and, other than the odd text, has not been able to talk to any of the other mothers about what has happened over the last fortnight. I can understand, and being of a somewhat less jovial disposition when it comes to engaging with other grown-ups at school, I'm happy to take the first shift and go home for the next couple of days. It's not easy – far from it – but the need to maintain a normal disposition is important as far as the outside world is concerned. This isn't because of what other people may or may not think, I don't care about that; but because of what Ellie, Luca and Millie think, and I care about that a lot.

I arrange to meet the headmaster tomorrow morning – the first day back at school. He had sent a reply to my initial call and email about Millie a few days ago. The school's support is also unequivocal – 'whatever it takes' to make our lives easier.

## 5) Day 12 – 4:30pm, Tuesday 16th April

The journey back to Tunbridge Wells allows me time to reflect on events. I would learn to welcome and appreciate these train journeys up and down from GOSH – small interludes of calm amid the rough and choppy sea we're currently crossing. I update my notes on the iPad (that I would later use for this diary) and research visual impairment and visual aids (a recent hobby of mine, for obvious reasons…).

As I get nearer to home, I start rehearsing the conversation I need to have with my eldest, Ellie Rose. Luca, who is four, I'm not so worried about. He won't get it, and he's been with his sister and aunty/mama, who he loves, all this time. Ellie is nine though, and was very close to Millie before all this happened, so I know she will be affected. She had never been without me or Vanessa for longer than a day and night before this – and she has now been without us for eleven days and eleven nights. That in itself is unusual, and although she was staying with her much-loved aunty and grand-parents, she is bound to have been affected by this unfamiliar turn of events. She is probably not aware of the more sinister implications of what has befallen Millie, but I'm sure she senses the seriousness of the situation nonetheless. Her expectations, worries and concerns therefore need to be managed. At the same time, she is also deserving of respect and truth as a full member of this family.

As part of the support provided by GOSH for parents in our situation, various leaflets have come our way, including those for charities that produce real-hair wigs (we bought one for £600 straight away but never used it. For children, hats are better – don't waste your money on wigs); helping your child to eat (chemotherapy suppresses appetite and can change children's taste); the 'little white book of brain tumour' support resources (not kidding); a parent's guide to childhood cancer; childhood brain and spinal cord tumour; welcome to Lion and Elephant Ward leaflet (the names of the two chemotherapy wards at GOSH – this has a smiling elephant and lion on the front – it doesn't manage to cheer me up); and also how to help brothers and sisters.

The only one I have found of real use is a children's book called *Mary Has a Brain Tumour*. I read through it, and it's our story, except for a few minor details. Mary is five, and is like any other little girl before she falls ill with what turns out to be a brain tumour. The book talks about what Mary has to go through, the tests she has to undertake, the operation, chemotherapy, her hair falling out, the radiotherapy. It's all there, including Mary's surprise at the end when she is cured: a little kitten (we even promised Millie a kitten when all this is finished. Oh dear, we parents are a predictable bunch…). It doesn't entirely reflect reality, but then it shouldn't. It's targeted at children, so all the characters in the book are smiling on every page and during each phase of each treatment. Even the kitten at the end is smiling.

We don't know how our story will end, of course, but as far as telling Ellie is concerned, my aim is clear; to get her acquainted with terminology she will hear at school (words like 'tumour', 'cancer', 'chemotherapy'). And to inform her of Millie's specific illness: it is cancer, but there are several types of cancer, not just one. Some cancer kills, absolutely, but some cancer can be cured. Millie's cancer is the kind that can be cured. That's all there is to it.

It will take time and effort. It may seem like a very high mountain to climb, a mountain whose top we cannot even begin to make out, lost as it is among obscure clouds of uncertainty; but as we struggle up the steep and narrow path, we know the hike looks worse from the bottom. We are determined to keep going, to put one arduous step in front of the other, before the light of the sun disappears behind the horizon.

*6) Day 12 – 6pm, Tuesday 16th April*

I finally get home and see Luca and Ellie for the first time since this all started. It's good to see them – their faces, their smiles and their ability to hug like healthy children. Seeing them only further emphasises how far Millie has fallen during the last fortnight, and how ill she really is. I feel sad for her. There is so much uncertainty at the moment, it is difficult to conceptualise what her life will be like, if she will have a life at all. Luca is clearly pleased to see me, Ellie a little less so. Daddy coming home means no more sleepovers at Mama and Josie's house. It is also clear that Ellie is old enough to have understood how unusual the situation is. I am sure she is concerned about Millie in some way, though she doesn't know it, and she is certainly unable to verbalise it, aged just nine. I will try to tread with care.

I put Luca to bed and go into Ellie's bedroom to have 'the chat' about Millie. I have the *Mary Has a Brain Tumour* book in my hand, but before we read it, I feel it is important to explain the situation using my own words. So I recount the last fortnight, I tell Ellie that Millie has a lump in her head that was making her feel sick, and that affected her eyes. I tell her Millie was very brave during her operation and will now have some special medicine to make sure we get rid of the nasty lump for good. Millie must stay in hospital for a while, so Mummy and Daddy will alternate between hospital and being at home for about the next three months. I mention the word cancer because I feel she needs to be equipped with a vocabulary she may encounter at school, or when she hears grown-ups talking. I reassure her that, while there are many different types of cancer, some very nasty indeed, the one Millie has can be cured. I also tell her how proud Mummy and Daddy are of her, of how helpful she has been over the last twelve days in looking after Luca Jack, and generally being really great away from home.

She seems to take the whole thing well, though clearly the upheaval has had an effect. She is disproportionately sad not to be at Mama's anymore and sends emotional messages on her iTouch to Jonny and Josie telling them she loves them and misses them. I let her stay up late with me and we have a bowl of noodles in the kitchen together. She decides to sleep with me tonight, and Luca also joins us in the middle of the night.

As I fall asleep with Ellie by my side, I reflect on Millie and her condition, on her first day of chemotherapy, on how her body and mind will react to the next few months of gruelling treatment. She is so young to be afflicted by such a violent disease (and equally violent a cure). I wish I could change that; I wish I could take on cancer myself and go through it on her behalf. I know it's not possible. Like the dead who cannot be profited by the prayers of the living, I know wishful thinking cannot benefit Millie. Only my focus on doing the right thing for me and my family can, only the tangible investment of my time, of Vanessa's time, and of the time of consultants and doctors at GOSH, who are doing their utmost to save her life.

# NOW WAS THE HOUR THAT
# WAKENS FOND DESIRE

*7) Day 13 – Wednesday 17th April*

First day of summer term – time to get up and get ready for school. The start of the summer term has come at the right time in the context of what is happening to us. It will prove an invaluable distraction for Ellie Rose, like a flowery valley in the middle of recent and future disruptions, as darkness hinders our daily lives.

I always thought I would feel a degree of apprehension at facing other grown-ups unconnected to family or the medical profession, post-cancer diagnosis. In particular, mums and dads and teachers from school, all so intimately involved with Millie over the last few years. I knew there would be much tilting of heads, of seemingly reassuring words of comfort and support. In a somewhat peculiar way, I actually feel for them having to face me, the father of a daughter recently diagnosed with a malignant brain tumour. I understand it is difficult for them to say the right thing, so I deliberately decide to be as pleasant and friendly as I can – to be supportive of their efforts to try and comfort what cannot be comforted. I also feel that, as far as this extended circle of acquaintances is concerned, they have a right to know and be informed. Millie has shared time with their children. They have a genuine interest and desire to be helpful. And some will actually be so incredibly, so exceedingly helpful, in so many ways, it is difficult to know how we will ever be able to thank them for it and the support they gave us during some very difficult times. Equally I am also determined to protect Luca, and Ellie in particular, by minimising recent events. Above all else, regardless of what others may think, my children need to feel their father is in control, that this situation is serious, of course, but nothing that will disrupt the daily routine of school, or indeed my mood and disposition.

I thought I'd feel emotional about seeing other parents, but I feel nothing. Compared with having to deal with the news of a malignancy diagnosis, this is child's play. In my desire to adopt a functional approach to help Millie, I have deliberately numbed my emotions to such a degree that I find the school run and updating mums and dads easy to handle. I even get unexpected hugs from mothers I have hardly spoken to before. Many come and tell me how sorry they are to hear our news, and I see genuine sorrow in their eyes.

It makes me think that our situation must seem unfathomably difficult to cope with by the outside world. We are now thirteen days into this nightmare, and the learning curve has been steep. It has required an extraordinary mental effort to adopt a functional attitude in order to operate, but so far we have been successful at 'holding it together'. I think that's all that can be expected at this early stage. I don't feel brave or courageous. We didn't choose to be the parents of a child with cancer, it happened to us, so we need to adapt fast, not for us but for our children; for Millie in particular. I know this is just the beginning, that Millie's affliction will require a long-term sustained effort. In the end, that may get to me too. We'll cross that bridge when we come to it. *One shot at a time.*

I take Ellie and Luca to their respective classes and go to see the headmaster, Mr M. I had never really spoken to Mr M at any length before, about anything. It is odd that the first real conversation I have with Mr M is to recount recent events, and for the first time out loud. For some reason, there is little emotion in my tone and I am able to narrate Millie's story somewhat matter-of-factly. We agree that the priority over the next few months is no longer the curriculum (all of a sudden maths and English don't seem so important...) and that the focus will be to ensure we preserve Millie's confidence and sense of belonging. This will involve reintegrating her into class at the start of the new school year. She is now in Year 2, so will rejoin her classmates in September for Year 3. Actually, this ends up being in November, but the principle will hold.

It is difficult to plan for Millie at the moment – this will be a long uncertain journey. Her eyesight is poor (she can barely make anything out, let alone read words on a page or a white board). She may well need special support or a school equipped to help children with her condition. She still has a lump in her brain that will need to be removed, she still has cancer and we don't know if chemotherapy will be successful in melting away the malignant cells. We agree it's too soon to make definite plans, but Mr M and the school's support is unequivocal – 'whatever it takes'.

More than the academic achievements, more than the sporting excellence, more than the idyllic, privileged setting in which education is dished out in daily doses – it is this spirit of solidarity, the genuine aim to be the best school it can be for Millie, Ellie and Luca (and us as parents) that makes me proud to be a parent at this institution (Speech Day and prize giving excluded).

*8) Day 14 – Thursday 18th April*

It's my turn to go up to GOSH this morning and stay with Millie for a couple of days and nights, while Ness comes home for two days. It's a routine we will perform over the next four months as Millie undergoes four cycles of chemotherapy and two further brain operations. I drop Ellie and Luca at school and take the train up to London. It's nice to see Millie again, even though I only left her a couple of days ago. She looks so unwell compared to the other two. She recognises me when I'm at the door though, and she has done a drawing of a blue butterfly and snail in a garden with a couple of trees. It's not perfect but the positioning of the snail, butterfly and trees clearly indicates she can see the page. The butterfly's left wing is somewhat detached from the body, but it's something. Actually, it's more than something. 'Improvement begets further improvement'. Like a celestial falcon, green as the tender leaves and newly born, this blue butterfly, for the first time since her loss of vision, gives me tangible hope for the continued recovery of her eyesight.

Unfortunately, that hope will quickly be quashed by the results of the electro-retinogram, which confirms severe impairment of the optic nerves (irreversible). Electroretinography is a test to measure the electrical response of the eye's light-sensitive cells. Results suggest that enough light is going through the optic nerves to possibly enable some functional recovery of eyesight, but nothing spectacular. It looks increasingly likely that Millie will be severely visually-impaired for the rest of her life. So much so that we are given details on how to apply for a blue badge, enabling us to park in areas designated for handicapped people.

The thought of having a seven-year-old child with cancer, and probably permanently severely visually-impaired is tough to handle. I suppress the emotions that try and come to the surface: sorrow, deep sadness for Millie – this young thing who was bouncing about only three weeks ago, and whose life will now be changed forever, probably for the worse. I kill those thoughts and go back to functional mode. It's the only way I know how to *be* at the moment.

I distract myself with her willingness to play some games. A couple of days back, I'd gone to Peter Jones just off Sloane Square, bought a suitcase and filled it with toys from the toy department. Anything I thought Millie might enjoy given her limited vision. Anything musical (Bop It), anything tactile (Play-Doh) and anything she used to enjoy before she got ill (Connect Four being a favourite). Connect Four would become a defining feature of the next few days as she was seeing enough to be able to play. I'd let her win most of the time, of course, as she couldn't quite see the whole grid, but she could see enough to pick a coin of the right colour and put it in the appropriate slot. Her depth perception was still poor, but once she'd tested the distance a couple of times, her hands would become more assured. She couldn't concentrate for very long, just a couple of games at a time, but I took what I could.

I enjoyed those little moments with Millie – those moments that enabled me to catch a few glimpses of the Millie of old, like bright stars near the North Pole. She was still there somewhere, lost and scared in the wretched depths of cancer, that serpent creeping subtly into the inner valleys of her brain. And I was determined to go and find her, or at least what remained of Millie, to grab her hand and take her back to a life she would find rich and fulfilling.

*9) Day 15 – Friday 19th April*

I wake up tired from the night, but tell myself that however bad my night might have been, it pales in comparison to what Millie is going through. I don't find being in hospital particularly difficult from the point of view of sleeplessness: just exceedingly wearisome on several other levels. Millie's lack of sight limits daily activities significantly (watching movies and TV programmes is not possible, for example), and there's only so much reading one can do. She is still very weak from her operation and finds it difficult to get up, so doesn't feel like going anywhere like the playroom. I can't leave Millie on her own other than to go and buy myself a quick sandwich, so being confined to this room, this ward, without the possibility to go and get some air is not the easiest of tasks. Again, however tough for me, it is a million-fold tougher for Millie.

My sister comes to visit me in hospital. I hadn't seen her for about a year. I appreciate her coming over, and find it comforting to see her. She has brought a variety of gifts for Millie, including the biggest teddy I have ever seen (though Millie thinks it's a Hello Kitty doll – so eyesight is still not quite there). We haven't seen each other much over the past ten years, but I find it soothing to have her there, to talk about old times, about my parents, about her own two children and about Millie. The conversation is somewhat tentative, unsure of itself and at times forced, hindered by a decade of virtual silence. But talking to her, however awkward, is helping me and I take it at face value. I am grateful to her for making the effort and for doing the right thing.

Talking to busy consultants and doctors is not easy either, in any hospital, and GOSH is no different. This is especially true during the first couple of weeks, as you get accustomed to the way things are done. Many leaflets are handed out but there's not much specific information about my daughter. Today, I receive the first official piece of correspondence from GOSH in the form of a letter, oddly not addressed to me, but to my local GP in East Sussex. It is from Dr H, Millie's consultant paediatric oncologist. A copy of it is sent to several people, including: the consultant ophthalmologist who saw us at Moorfields the day after diagnosis; Dr D, Millie's paediatrician; Dr S, consultant paediatric endocrinologist (though we would end up using another consultant endocrinologist at GOSH); and Dr P, consultant paediatrician at Pembury (our local hospital – where we ended up spending more time then we imagined at this stage of treatment); and last but by no means least, my wife and me. That's a lot of people, and a relatively old-fashioned way of communicating (it must have a value, but I haven't yet discovered what that is). I presume doctors also communicate by email, but choose this more formal approach for discharge letters and other documents recording milestones in Millie's illness. Her file, which was a slim blue folder when we first arrived, is gathering inches by the day.

Anyway, back to the letter and its content. Firstly, it confirms the diagnosis – that of a 'Supersellar tumour, consistent with a secreting germ cell tumour' – and the fact she has a raised serum tumour and Beta-hCG – both of which are tumour markers in the blood, indicating malignancy. Secondly, it describes the presenting problems: 1) Excessive thirst consistent with diabetes insipidus – 12–18 months. That's about right. 2) Three-week history of headaches and sudden loss of vision three days prior to diagnosis (that's not entirely accurate – Millie had a couple of headaches that went as quickly as they came about four weeks before all this started). Thirdly, the letter summarises the treatment: 1) Emergency debulking surgery to decompress optic nerves. 2) Commenced PEI (cisplatin, etoposide and ifosfomide chemotherapy), according to the intracranial germ cell tumour guidelines.

Up until today, I think the worst correspondence I had ever received was a redundancy email from a large accountancy firm, the day after my return from honeymoon (so caring). Nothing compared to this though.

Just a few lines to recount the single most traumatic event of my life, my family's life and my daughter's life. I read on. The letter briefly describes Millie, how she was when she arrived a fortnight ago, some of the presenting problems, including what we thought was blurred vision, and what turned out to be blindness. It summarises Dr H's discussions with us about the provisional diagnosis from the tumour markers: 'That of a rare malignant (cancerous) tumour known as a secreting intracranial germ cell tumour... these tumours are very rare, with fewer than ten cases a year in the UK'. We are still awaiting the histopathology at this point. The letter has one piece of good news in the whole three pages: 'Initial CSF cytology do not show any metastatic lesions. Therefore she has localised tumour, which is standard risk'. Oh goody – standard risk. Jokes aside, had the tumour spread, it would have significantly reduced her chances of survival to about one in five. And then the meaningless sentence on prognosis: 'Multimodality treatment sees over

65% progression-free survival reported in children', before ensuring expectations are firmly set: 'Although, of course, this does mean that some children relapse and the chance of cure second time round is greatly reduced'. Best not to think about that then – not yet. In any event, if there is one area that severely lacks any meaningful information, it is that which covers progression-free survival.

Progression-free survival is the one question parents most want to know the answer to (will my daughter live or will she die?). The second most important question is often impossible to answer. And that's 'If she does live, what sort of quality of life can she expect, given the aggressive nature of the treatment she will undergo, and the material sequelae she is likely to have both as a result of cancer and of the cure'.

Finally, the letter touches on the concept of shared care. This is something we are not entirely familiar with, but there will be plenty of time and occasions to learn about it. It basically means we have a local hospital that will provide support during the times we are at home, in between chemotherapy treatments.

It's the first time I have read something formal from GOSH specifically relating to Millie and what's been happening to her – and with a medical summary of the last fortnight. The tangible quality of this correspondence cements the morbid and sinister nature of her condition. It makes it far more real and it takes me a while to regroup.

I read it again in the night when I'm alone, resting on the small bed provided for parents, next to where Millie is sleeping. I read it in disbelief, wondering, doubting, bewildered and confused, as if carried up the mountain we need to climb in the coming months, asleep and dreaming: dreaming of a cure, of better days to come. In the hour that awakens fond desires, such dreams, burdened by darkness of the most unspeakable kind, are incapable of surfacing. I'm tired. I need to sleep. Tomorrow is another day.

# WHEN WE HAD PASSED THE THRESHOLD OF THE GATE

*10) Day 16 – Saturday 20th April*

The letter with the 65% statistic plays on my mind (two in three children live, one in three dies). Researching on the internet for this type of cancer is not an easy task. There is too much information not specific enough to be of any value. There are 332,000 results on Google, much of it relating to all types of secreting germ cell tumours, not just those found in the confines of the skull. It's such a rare form of cancer that it doesn't really feature in any of the regular literature describing brain tumours. When it does, it's far too general and superficial to be of any value. Staging is also quite confusing, as the system appears to vary according to the type of tumour. Millie's is a mature teratoma ('terato' from ancient Greek, meaning monster and 'oma' as a suffix-forming noun indicating disease). Millie literally has a monster disease. Indeed she has.

I find very little in terms of studies, pilot studies and cooperative projects between countries. Nothing that says, 'We looked at one hundred children with this affliction and sixty-five of them survived five years, and sixty-five of them looked and felt like normal eighteen-year-olds further down the line'. Remember there are two questions every parent wants to know: will my child live? And if she does, what will life be like for her? Both questions are difficult to answer when they relate to individual cases. They can only be answered generally in the context of the vague, ambiguous rhetoric of consultants.

If there is one area where improvement could be made in NHS hospitals, it is the way in which communication happens – even in one of the best, if not *the* best hospital in the UK. Communication is not frequent enough, access to the right information is poor, connectivity within the hospital itself is non-existent for patients and parents of patients, and the vast quantity of data gathered about my daughter here (daily blood and other tests, opinions gathered at weekly consultants' meetings etc.) are simply not available, in any form, to parents. The only information comes in the form of old-fashioned letters after significant events or on discharge, and the irregular visits made by consultants.

What's more, in the age of information and communication, I have not yet been given a single email address, most phone numbers go to a switch board of some kind or another, and secretaries are difficult to reach (other than Amy and Emily – you know who you are – I thank you for your contactability and professionalism). If you want to speak to the lead consultant, you have to go through three strata of human beings; from nurses to registrars to doctors on call. More often than not, you have to wait until the next day to get a reply that ought to be simpler and more effective to deliver – most definitely an area for improvement.

Fast forward a few months to the USA, where Millie will undergo proton beam therapy – more on that later – and the chasm in technology and communication smacks you in the face. All hospitals have guest Wi-Fi, so you can log in to your daughter's medical records, and you are given a book filled with business cards of the nurses and doctors who will look after you, with email addresses, direct lines and mobile numbers. I will talk more about the difference in culture in Part III of this book.

Back to the scrolls and parchments of the NHS... This is Millie's last day of her first chemotherapy cycle, though not her last day in hospital. So though we have passed this first threshold of the gate, we are not out of Elephant Ward yet. Following the first onslaught of chemotherapeutic drugs, and the vast amount of liquid that's been pumped into her system, coupled with deficiencies in certain hormones due to the tumour damaging the pituitary, we can't go home yet. Millie is not stable, so we need to stay for another few days. How many, we do not yet know. Hospitals, and this type of illness, certainly have a way of keeping you humble, and we would encounter many stories of humility along the way, far greater than our own. But now it's time to go back to East Sussex and for Vanessa to come up to do her shift.

*11) Day 21 – Thursday 25th April*

Four days after finishing Millie's first bout of chemotherapy, nineteen days after diagnosis, we are finally initiating the process of discharge. It will be the first time since 6th April that we will have left the hospital to go home, and it will probably happen tomorrow. One malignant brain tumour, an eight-hour craniotomy and a first cycle of chemotherapy later, we are finally getting ready to go back home. Millie is very weak at this stage. This first chemical onslaught has been extremely hard on her seven-year-old body, and she has needed five days to re-stabilise from an endocrinological and fluid perspective.

Being sent home brings with it a degree of apprehension. Millie is now on four daily medications, all of which have been administered by nurses so far. They are:

- **DDAVP** (desmopressin): A modified form of the normal human hormone arginine vasopressin, which limits the amount of water eliminated in urine. This medication is given as a result of Millie's diabetes insipidus (damage to the specific cells in her pituitary gland that produce the hormone in the first place, or, more specifically, it is derived from a chemical that is synthesised in the hypothalamus and stored in the posterior pituitary). Millie needs to take desmopressin three times a day to mimic the way in which arginine vasopressin is released naturally in the body. DDAVP comes in 100 microgram tablets and she needs 10 micrograms three times a day (i.e. a miniscule dose of active ingredient). This means crushing a tablet, diluting it with 5ml of water, mixing it all up and extracting 0.5ml, using a 1.0ml syringe. It occurs to me that the margin of error with such doses must be quite high, and having three stages to the preparation (crushing, diluting and extracting) probably compounds the error rate so that Millie never actually gets 10mg three times a day, but probably somewhere between 8 and 12.
- **Hydrocortisone:** In a few days we will switch to hydrocortisone. For the time being she is being weaned off dexamethasone, a strong steroid that was initially given to her when she was first diagnosed in order to reduce the swelling caused by the tumour. Hydrocortisone belongs to a group of medicines called corticosteroids (referred to

simply as steroids). It is used as a replacement treatment for people whose adrenal glands do not produce enough natural corticosteroid. Corticosteroid, or cortisol more specifically, is produced in the adrenal cortex by the adrenal glands, just above the kidneys, and is involved in a wide range of physiological processes, including stress response, immune response, and the regulation of inflammation and carbohydrate metabolism. The trigger for cortisol production happens in the hypothalamus (secretion of corticotropin-releasing hormone – CRH), which in turn triggers cells in the pituitary to secrete another hormone, adrenocorticotropic hormone (ACTH). Blood carries it to the adrenal cortex and stimulates the adrenals to produce cortisol. Millie is given hydrocortisone preventatively because dexamethasone suppresses the production of ACTH, which in turns suppresses the ability of the adrenal glands to produce cortisol. While Millie is taking hydrocortisone, the adrenals cease to work, thus starting a vicious circle of hormonal deficiencies which broadly means we don't know if her adrenal glands can be jump-started back to life again (or indeed if Millie will eventually be able to produce ACTH of her own). This is a complex area, which we will revisit later, as hydrocortisone is a ghastly substance whose dreadful side effects make millions suffer every day. Back to Millie, who will be taking 10mg daily, three times a day (5mg in the morning, 2.5mg after lunch and 2.5mg in the evening before bedtime). As it comes in 10mg tablets, we are using three tablets a day and going through the same process we employ to dilute DDAVP.

- **Ranitidine:** Given to counter one of the side effects of hydrocortisone (too much acid being produced in the stomach, causing stomach ulcers). This she takes twice a day, once in the morning and once in the evening – it comes in liquid form and she takes 60mg (or 4ml in a syringe).

- **Levothyroxine**: The easiest of the four to administer. This is a thyroid hormone (T4) produced by the cells of the thyroid gland and regulated by TSH (thyroid-stimulating hormone) made by – yup, you've guessed it – the pituitary gland. It may be that Millie's low levels of T4 are due to the tumour damaging the pituitary gland or it may be hereditary, as Vanessa is on levothyroxine post-pregnancy. And much in the same way as all these hormones seem to work, once you replace it, the body loses its ability to re-stimulate production, so she will be on it for life. Millie will need to take 50mg daily, and arithmetic and practicality are on our side this time, as it comes in small 50mg tablets that she has no difficulty swallowing.

All of these medicines Millie will have to take for the rest of her life (hopefully long life – we don't know at this stage). I mentioned briefly in the first part of this book how I feel about these additional restrictions. I have come to terms with probably the most difficult element of it – there is no, or very little, choice if she is going to have some quality of life in the long term. And this is subject to being cured of cancer, which is by no means a certainty at this stage. The alternative is no quality of life, or no life for that matter. In the same way we *all* need to eat and drink every single day to live, Millie will have a few extra things she needs to integrate as part of her daily routine. We are lucky to live in an age where science has enabled the manufacture of substances that replicate what the body produces. Up until about fifty years ago, vasopressin, for example, could not be synthesised artificially, so had to be extracted from deceased people.

In addition to all this, we are given a hydrocortisone emergency kit. This is in case Millie experiences symptoms of extreme weakness and a serious drop in blood pressure and mental confusion as a result of cortisol insufficiency (if she misses a couple of doses of hydrocortisone she will not be very well – far from it). If this happens, she will need extra steroid medication immediately, and may need an emergency injection. The kit consists of an injection of 100mg hydrocortisone sodium, so the little bag includes syringes, needles and the steroid liquid. We are not trained on how to administer it (oddly…), we are just told to take it with us wherever we go, call an ambulance in the event of an emergency and give them the kit to administer to Millie. Sounds overly complex for a simple injection, but the overload of information at this stage is such that challenging the medical profession (or the chemist going through all this) just doesn't come to mind. We are also given a card that says Millie is on hydrocortisone and if required can collect some at any pharmacy in the UK. In time, she may have to wear a bracelet or a necklace to let people know of her condition. And, finally, an emergency kit in case the Hickman lines get yanked out of her body. A little bag is provided containing antiseptic wipes, injection caps, flushing supplies, clamps and antibiotic ointment.

At this stage all this material, all these drug taking necessities are overwhelming, but in time we learn to cope with the requirement to administer medication with relative ease. There is so much information coming our way that it is difficult to consider a life at home on our own, without nurses to give the right doses at the right time. We haven't been told about shared care yet; the role our local hospital and local nursing team will play in the next few months.

So no biggie really, and no point feeling sorry for us or Millie for all this 'medicine taking'. The fact remains that she will have to lug the burden of daily pills for the rest of her life. But these rocks will not hinder her progress, and that's where we can help at these initial stages. The only thing to do is to make sure we are structured enough to administer the right doses at the right time. And that I feel certain we can be compliant with.

## 12) Day 22 – Friday 26th April

Today is a huge day for Millie and for us as a family – we are finally going home after twenty straight days in hospital. Millie is well enough to be discharged, though we know much still needs to be achieved and many hurdles overcome. She has another three chemotherapy cycles to go – we have only done one and it hasn't been easy – and at least one more brain operation (it will be two more in the end), before receiving some form of radiotherapy over six to eight weeks. It's the end of April now and we figure we're in it until the end of August (how wrong we were with that initial estimate! It seems the planning fallacy also applies to personal challenges).

The GOSH pharmacist goes through the dosages of the bag of medicines we are taking away with us. I tidy the room we have lived in for the last two weeks, and wait for Vanessa's brother, Jonny, who is coming to collect us and driving us down to East Sussex in his father's comfortable car. Millie is still very weak, but she is managing to get in and out of bed by herself (sort of) to go to the toilet and back, still holding on to the side of her bed as she does so. Not being hooked up to two big IV pumps helps (it wasn't fun doing that every twenty minutes for a couple of weeks). She's generally quite flat. Her concentration level is very poor (five minutes of anything is generally enough at this stage, before she asks to have a rest). Walking has been a struggle, especially as she can't see beyond a couple of metres at the moment, and we are still none the wiser as to whether it will improve. I am not hopeful (thankfully, on this one, I will be proved spectacularly wrong). But then what did we expect? She has cancer and has just begun one of the most gruelling treatments anyone can ever go through. It's tough to cope with as an adult, let alone as a child.

Millie's happy to come home, though it's hard to 'read' her at the moment. The last two weeks have changed her considerably, and I realise it will take a long time to rebuild what cancer and curing cancer has destroyed and will continue to demolish over the coming months. I glance down at her, her face like those of carved stone images on tombs that depict the dead inside. Sadness fills me to see Millie so changed, so irrevocably, so irreversibly. I only hope she will not endure too much suffering both physically in the short term and mentally in the long term. I try not to think ahead. *One shot at a time.* The next one is about getting her home and surviving the next three weeks out of hospital, ready for her second cycle of chemotherapy. The first is already having an effect on her blood count; but more on that later.

It takes the whole day to get discharged from GOSH, as everyone needs to sign off their respective part (endocrine, oncology, doctors, registrars, pharmacists double checking doses and medicines – and so on). We finally walk out at around 6pm, just in time for Friday rush hour out of London. I curse the NHS for taking a whole fucking day, when we had tried so hard to plan this for the last four days. I have since learned there is little point getting upset about the inefficiencies and intricacies of NHS discharges – you just can't fight it. By the end of the fourth session of chemotherapy, I had all the medicines I needed at home anyway, so I would give nurses and doctors deadlines to speed things up a little (i.e. "There is little point in waiting for medicines I already have. If the pharmacist is not ready by x o'clock, I'll just pick my stuff up and go home."). The journey back home is comfortable and Millie even plays one of her new favourite games – 'I spy', by some twisted logic. I think it provides her with some reassurance that she can still see something, and I also feel she wants us to know she can still see something, as if all this is her fault and she is trying to make us feel better about it. My heart weeps at the thought. It takes us a good three hours to get home, but we get there. Finally, Millie is *home* again.

Vanessa is waiting at the door, as is Ellie – looking nervous. Millie goes and sits on the sofa in the kitchen. Millie is home. It's quite surreal. We can't quite believe how much we've gone through over the last fortnight, how much is still to be achieved and how much uncertainty remains. Millie is home. We take her up to bed. She falls asleep. We decide it's best that one of us sleeps with her in her bed tonight, just in case.

I soon join Millie and as I listen to the sound of her slow, steady breathing, I fall asleep beside her. There is nowhere else I want to be in the world at this moment in time. Millie is home.

But not for long, as it turns out.

# OH PLEASANT LIGHT, MY
# CONFIDENCE AND HOPE!

*13) Day 23 – Saturday 27th April*

Millie wakes up feeling unwell – she has had an adequate night but has a temperature of 38.2°C. Not huge, but over 38°C. We were told this might happen, though not so soon, and that protocol dictates that any temperature over 38°C (two readings, one hour apart) has to be treated preventatively with antibiotics. The reason for this is that Millie is on her way to neutropenia (now here's another word I was not aware of when this all started). This is an abnormally low level of neutrophils, a type of white blood cell. All white blood cells help the body fight infection. Neutrophils fight infection by destroying harmful bacteria and fungi such as yeast that invade the body. People who have neutropenia are at increased risk of developing serious infection because they don't have enough neutrophils to destroy the harmful microorganisms that cause disease. Antibiotics are given preventatively whenever a fever appears so as to avoid infections occurring, because the body does not have any defensive mechanism left.

Millie would become neutrapenic about ten days after every chemotherapy session, with her level of neutrophils going down to nearly zero. Blood count analysis includes not just neutrophils, but also white blood cells, platelets (responsible for clotting) and red blood count. All of these will take a battering over the four chemotherapy cycles she will undergo in the next three months. So much so that she will need a transfusion of both platelets and red blood cells every time, at least once, sometimes twice in between treatments. At the lowest level of neutrophils, Millie will, we have been told, most likely develop an infection and have to go to hospital to be given antibiotics preventatively. Her neutrophil count would then start to rise again as her bone marrow resumes normal production. It may take three to four weeks to return to normal level, and slower and slower after each of the treatments. This is the main reason for chemotherapy sessions being spread as they are (one week on, three weeks off). Treatment does not start until the blood count has recovered sufficiently to be assaulted again by chemical agents. I don't think we'll be having much fun over the next three months. And I'm right. It won't be fun – for Millie in particular.

So back to the temperature; we phone Hedgehog Ward, the children's ward at Pembury Hospital, a brand-new NHS facility on our doorstep. In that respect we are lucky, as we would spend some time in this hospital both as an inpatient and, more frequently, as an outpatient. They know who we are as GOSH's referral letter has gone to them. What Millie has is so rare and exceptional, she is one of very few with this condition in the local area, if not the only one. Remember, only ten a year in the UK have her specific tumour. It is reassuring to know we are in the system – that the hospital is aware of us, of Millie, and that they can advise us about the right course of action.

The hospital tells us what we don't want to hear – that we

have to go in. One night at home, and we know we'll be spending at least another few days in our local hospital. No point in feeling sorry for ourselves, and no time. We know it is the right thing to do, so I pack a few things and take Millie in. Vanessa stays with Luca and Ellie for the time being, but being so close to home, we know it will be logistically easier to alternate nights at Pembury. We've been to this hospital a few times before – to A&E in particular. I had pneumonia a couple of years back and Ellie had a suspected fracture in her arm after falling off the monkey bars at school. It is an incredible facility, white and imposing, clean, efficient.

The ward itself is expecting us, we are taken to the assessment room, where a nurse comes to take blood for analysis, this time bacterial culture – to see if Millie has an infection. As it's Saturday, and this is not London, we won't have the results until Tuesday. In the meantime, they have to follow protocol and give Millie IV antibiotics preventatively. We're here for the night, that's for sure, and probably the next four to five days. On the plus side, the rooms are far superior in quality to GOSH and certainly more spacious, so that's something. The nurses resume control of the administration of Millie's medicines, which is a good thing – though in time, it will become a bad thing, as experience of our own daughter's condition will mean we will become much more adept at giving her the right dose at the right time than anyone else. Vanessa comes over and sets herself up to do the first night. I will do tomorrow afternoon and night.


*14) Day 24 – Sunday 28th April*


Millie is now starting to lose her hair following her first session of chemotherapy. It hadn't really happened until now, but big clumps are coming off whenever her hair is slightly pulled or brushed. She is aware of it, but probably doesn't have the energy to feel aggrieved. The current look isn't a great one, with ragged hair, witch-like bald patches and tufts of hair that haven't yet fallen out in other places. We knew this moment would come, we were oddly fearful of it without quite knowing why, but it's quite a hard one to swallow, even though we know the hair will grow back a couple of months after the last cycle has finished. It's an affirmation of the most dreaded illness one can get, and perhaps the most tangible evidence of what she is going through; the single most visible element of chemotherapy – she's got cancer, no question about it. You never tend to think about hair until your seven-year-old loses it. And it won't be just the hair on her head that Millie will lose. Eventually, with the second, third and fourth cycle she will lose most of her eyebrows and eyelashes.

Vanessa convinces Millie to cut her remaining hair short – might as well be done with it and not have to remove big bundles from her pillow every couple of hours. Mama brings a great hat to the hospital. Millie will have dozens of hats bought for her in time, but it is this first one she grows most accustomed to. It is her favourite by far and makes hair loss significantly more manageable for her, as well as for us. It's a white and pink kitty-cat hat with small fabric ears and a little beaded snout for a nose. The hat also becomes a talking point, allowing everyone we meet an easy conversation starter – that of complimenting the hat. It will transcend its practical purpose and make Millie feel special beyond the function it is there to perform. Never underestimate the power of a simple hat and its significance and assistance in the context of this illness, especially when children are concerned. Millie's illness must be obvious to outsiders (we got used to seeing her this way), but telling Millie what a *beautiful* hat she has is something 99% of all adults say when they meet us. It pleases me to see that side of humanity – how complete strangers feel instant empathy with a young girl afflicted with cancer.

During Millie's stay in Elephant Ward at GOSH, I had bought her a large TV with an integrated DVD player to put on her bed table. Given she could play Connect Four, I was hoping she would be able to see a screen close by. Unfortunately, her first choice of movie was *High School Musical*, and she was incapable of focusing on the fast-moving images. She gave up watching after a minute and was reluctant to try anything else for a while. Eventually she agreed to try something slightly gentler. I think it was *Little Princess*, and that actually worked, which was a blessing, given the state of her vision. In any case, I take the TV to Pembury hospital and with it an old *Dora the Explorer* game console (very simple, for 3+), but she seems able to play it and enjoys the experience of control she has from a hand/eye perspective. Over the next four days in Pembury, her vision would improve such that she would be able to see *Peppa Pig* on the wall-mounted television provided in each room.

It was here, in this room, on Sunday 28th April 2013, that I experienced one of the defining moments of my life so far. I had brought a few books about animals back from the playroom, with questions on each page, like: what do you call a group of lions? I was talking to Uncle Jonny, who had come to visit, and I was unaware that Millie, regaining confidence in her improving vision, had picked up one of the books. For the first time since 5th April, she started reading a sentence out loud. Jonny and I stopped talking, and lived one of those magical moments where time stands still. For five consecutive minutes, Millie, with increasing speed and a clear sense of achievement and excitement, picked up the books and read the titles on all the pages. She can read! She can read big print!

Oh pleasant light, my confidence and hope! Photons are clearly travelling through her optic nerves and bring with them the promise of further improvement.

Being in hospital for a possible bacterial infection matters little now. It's meant we've got accustomed with how to bring her here, and met some of the local doctors and nurses that would help us over the next few months. No infection was found, and we ended up going back home a couple of days later.


## 15) Day 29 – Friday 3rd May

Whilst under the care of GOSH for the treatment of her brain tumour, Millie (and us) will be assisted by a team of four community nurses. District or community nurses mainly visit patients at home. Their role includes supporting the patient and carer at home, administering treatments such as wound dressing (in Millie's case, the dressing covering her Hickman line, which needs replacing at least once a week), taking blood from her Hickman line, injections (none at the moment, but there will be some a few weeks down the line), monitoring health and offering general practical advice on aspects of healthcare at home for Millie.

We are visited today, for the first time, by one such nurse. She is great, and Millie takes to her immediately, which helps. She has some trouble taking blood from Millie's Hickman line, which can sometimes be temperamental, but thankfully always ends up working. Taking blood and analysing it plays a vital role in between chemotherapy sessions. Chemotherapy has a violent effect on blood count (red, white, neutrophils and platelets are all affected), so it is critical to take readings every couple of days. If the community nurse cannot come (on bank holidays or weekends) and blood is due to be taken, then we would go to our local hospital instead. These blood test results are then stored in her file, and GOSH reviews this weekly to establish when to start the next course of chemotherapy. Millie's neutrophils are beginning to show signs of life, so starting to recover. They told us this would happen but there is always an element of reassurance when the body does as it is expected to do.

Vanessa and I are still taking turns to sleep with her, and Millie is generally still weak from the cumulative assault of surgery and chemotherapy. We were warned that chemotherapy would be tough on her, and it is. Millie makes an effort to be up and about, and Vanessa takes her for short walks to the local church and back – not to go in and pray, it just happens to be a nice walk.

Still, the toxic substances that have been injected into her over five days have enveloped her in a fog, dark as night, depriving her and most of her cells of pure air.

# OTHER GOOD THERE IS, WHERE MAN FINDS NOT HIS HAPPINESS

*16) Day 33 – Tuesday 7th May*

Millie has now recovered sufficiently from a blood count perspective to start her second cycle of chemotherapy. Neither Vanessa nor I are looking forward to it, but neither of us will have to endure it first hand, so we pick ourselves up and tell ourselves to get on with it. After the lull of a few days spent at home amongst semblances of normality, it takes effort to be brought back to the reality of life caring for a cancer patient. We are only at the beginning of our journey, and we need to revert back to our usual functional approach. Once again we take turns, so Vanessa and her mother will travel to London with Millie this morning.

This time, she will be admitted to Lion Ward (the other oncology ward, next door to Elephant Ward). Same sort of ward, different nurses. This time, Millie was able to get involved with packing for hospital, which helped, as opposed to the last time we made this trip, when she was blind and undiagnosed. I spend a couple of days at home looking after the other two, then switch over with Vanessa to spend a couple of days at GOSH – and so on and so forth.

We know we are in for more of the same: five days of chemotherapy, with at least two to four days of re-stabilising Millie from an endocrinological perspective. PEI protocol will continue to apply so over five days she will be given cisplatin, etoposide and ifosfomide intravenously, 24/7. Cisplatin is so toxic it has the potential to injure and damage the kidneys, especially as it is given in combination with ifosfomide, which also affects kidneys – as well as cause hearing loss. We also know it's more of the same with endocrine measuring inputs and outputs, weighing her urine every time she goes to the loo, and keeping a record of all the liquid she drinks. The main monitoring relates to her diabetes insipidus for which she is taking a drug called desmopressin (DDAVP).

Much of the work of endocrine doctors is to measure her inputs versus outputs and ensure she maintains a healthy balance of both by giving the right dose at the right time. Neither would be achieved for much of the time we spend in hospital, but such is the obsession with sodium levels that most of my arguments at GOSH end up being with the various endocrine registrars who roam the wards in search of the next soul to torment. This fixation on sodium and a tendency to alter the dose of DDAVP by minute amounts seem to be limited to the realms of mid-level endocrine registrars. Consultants are happy to prescribe higher doses over the phone when we are at home, without once mentioning or measuring sodium.

Before Millie starts with the first wave of chemicals, the customary kidney function test is undertaken, to ensure her organs can sustain another ordered attack of poisonous substances given systematically over five days. She had one prior to her first course of treatment, one in between, and protocol dictates that one is performed before starting her second bout. The GFR (or glomerular filtration rate) test itself is pretty simple. A dye is injected into her blood stream and blood is taken at regular intervals to establish how efficient the kidneys are at eliminating it. Her kidneys are fine, though they won't be for long. She can start her second session. Here we go again.

Life on an oncology ward is surprisingly serene. Whilst chemotherapeutic agents are violent at the cellular level, their administration is somewhat ordered and calm. The nurses come in at regular intervals and hook Millie up with one drug or another – this then infuses for a number of hours, before another drug is put up. And so it continues throughout the day, with the only loud interruptions coming from the pumps themselves, beeping every time a drug runs out, or pressure builds in her veins: manageable during the day, less so during the night. The drugs themselves generally induce somnolence (they tell me they make you feel as though you have bad flu) so Millie, while uncomfortable, spends much of her time sleeping, day and night, interrupted only by the need to change her bed sheets. Diabetes insipidus, compounded by severe tiredness, double-compounded by seven litres of liquid going into your body a day, inevitably lead to a few wet beds. The nurses are used to it, however, and generally amazing at dealing with changing bed sheets and any mess caused by bodily fluids originating from any of the three main orifices.

Severe nausea was one of the side effects I'd mostly related to chemotherapy before all this started. Oddly, Millie is seldom sick. She is given a regular anti-sickness drug and is generally off food (who wouldn't be?), but other than that, little if no vomiting has occurred so far (we'll make up for that stroke of good fortune after her second operation, as if to restore the fundamental balance of the universe as far as luck is concerned).

The tranquillity of an oncology ward is deceiving – the toxins injected into Millie by the bucket are poisons, as we would shortly find out. And, as we are gently guided, like the blind, across the fields of biological warfare, the dark fog of hell would soon descend on us and Millie yet again.


## 17) Day 37 – Saturday 11th May

I was in East Sussex when it happened. Vanessa was with Millie at GOSH. It's the last day of the second cycle of chemotherapy, or Chemo Two, as we were now referring to the treatments and as if familiarity with them somehow makes them more casual – it doesn't. Millie had started swelling from pretty much everywhere, but hands and legs in particular, and her midriff. Initially, the intelligentsia at GOSH thought this might be related to desmopressin regulating the amount of fluid the kidneys were processing. Further digging revealed it was kidney failure; or, more specifically, acute kidney failure caused by one of the chemotherapeutic agents injected into her, most probably cisplatin, or the cumulative blitz of cisplatin and ifosfomide taken together.

*Acute kidney failure.* I repeat the words in my head without knowing the true implications. It sounds pretty serious (it is). I know kidneys are *vitally* important organs without which the body cannot function (cue dialysis machine). At worst, acute kidney failure can be fatal (oh good, something else that can kill Millie). It happens when your kidneys are suddenly unable to filter waste products from your blood. When kidneys lose

137

their filtering ability, dangerous levels of waste accumulate and the blood's chemical makeup gets out of balance. One quick and easy way to find out is via a blood test to measure creatinine levels. Creatinine is a byproduct of muscle metabolism and is removed from the blood chiefly by the kidneys, primarily by glomerular filtration (ah, that old chestnut again). A later GFR test (glomerular filtration rate test) would indeed confirm damage to the kidneys. Not just any damage – possibly irreversible damage. In other words, in the process of curing cancer, Millie's kidneys may have been permanently injured by the cytotoxic substances injected in her body. 'May', 'possibly', 'irreversibly'. Ambiguity in possible outcomes happens often in the course of the long journey one travels to cure cancer.

Now and again, cataclysmic events occur in the body, primarily as a result of attempting to cure the disease. These events can have devastating and life-changing consequences, and can damage perfectly healthy organs, such as the kidneys or ears, that were not directly threatened by the disease itself. Bad luck is compounded by the advanced (yet still parochial) way of treating this affliction.

Chemo Two is over, but Millie is really unwell. After spending a night being monitored every hour as a result of her kidney failure, she lies motionless for most of the day, bereft of energy – trapped on her misty mountain where sunlight still can't reach. She can barely walk and she can barely see, as the chemotherapy affects her eyes for reasons we have not yet been able to establish. It's probably to do with levels of energy and her ability to focus and concentrate – so short term only. She is as far removed from the young girl we knew as I could ever have imagined. And the road ahead has just been made more difficult by this latest episode. There is little that can be done other than wait and bring down her creatinine by further

IV flushing, so we know we're in it (or rather, Millie is) for another two to three days at least.

Oddly, when we eventually receive the discharge letter, it states in the first paragraph that Millie 'tolerated the chemotherapy reasonably well'. Hmmm... It then goes on to say (*in the same letter*) that she 'developed acute renal failure after her dose of cisplatin? Drug-related injury? Dehydration?' The question marks are in the letter, by the way. I have not added them myself for comedic effect.

Meanwhile, as part of the conversation taking place between Vanessa and Millie's oncologist, Dr H, Vanessa mentions proton beam therapy to him for the first time. Vanessa's sister, Josie, had sent her an article from the *Daily Mail* recounting the story of a young boy with a similar affliction to Millie, who was not accepted for funding under the NHS for Proton Beam radiotherapy and whose parents were trying to raise the money independently. Reading briefly about proton beam, it becomes clear it is a better type of radiation therapy for Millie because of its fewer side effects on cognition, compared to conventional radiotherapy (more on these types of therapy in Part III – Heaven). Vanessa and I have already had plenty of conversations about this and we are clear that with or without NHS funding (but still under the care and supervision of GOSH), we wanted the possibility of proton beam further down the line if it would indeed be the better form of therapy for Millie.

Dr H confirms that, actually, the possibility of proton beam had already been discussed at their weekly meeting (ah! News to us – no one at GOSH had mentioned proton beam to us before) and that Millie's radiation oncologist (oh good, another specialist) would cover it as part of the meeting we are due to have this coming Monday. Good thing Vanessa mentioned proton beam to Dr H in such a timely fashion.

I'm back in London. It's switch over day. This time, Vanessa stays on for a bit so that I can meet with Dr C, Millie's radiation oncologist. This is an important meeting as it will determine the initial plan for Millie following chemotherapy. Radiotherapy was always on the cards for this type of tumour – multimodality of treatment (as it's called) improves prognosis, and we were told Millie would have it when we met Dr H for the first time.

What we didn't know is that radiotherapy comes in several forms. One of these forms in particular has the benefits of fewer side effects because of the physics involved. This is called proton beam. From the information we have been able to gather, we think this type of radiation would be effective in Millie's case, so we're keen to explore the option further. Being a firm believer in always hearing the opinion of experts (the validity of which is to be challenged sometimes, no doubt), I have always felt that a) I wanted this view confirmed by someone who knows about it; and b) I wanted them to understand that if this was the right choice, NHS funding or not, I wanted Millie to have it, but clearly if not funded, I still wanted to remain under the watchful eye of GOSH. I believed then – as I believe now – that they have always had the best interests of Millie at heart. Not because she was Millie, or special in any way, or my daughter, but because she was a patient under their care.

I wait for Dr C up in Safari Ward. This is the oncology day ward where children come for their fix of chemotherapy if they do not require hospitalisation. It's another reminder that Millie hasn't had it easy, though there will also be plenty of reminders that she's been pretty lucky compared to others.

I don't just see Dr C. As I enter the room, there are two or three other doctors and students of various categories. I wear my humble hat – the best one to wear when you want strangers to like you. I am asked to recall the story so far and I do; the diabetes insipidus, the loss of vision, the first MRI scan revealing a tumour, the first operation, the first two cycles of chemotherapy, the acute kidney failure, the potential growth hormone deficiency. I explain my position with regards to proton beam and Dr C confirms that, yes, while the chances of local control and therefore cure would be equivalent with protons or conventional photon radiotherapy, there *may* be *some decrease* in the cognitive sequelae with proton radiotherapy. So, just like photon radiotherapy, there's no certainty with regards to cure, but possibly, maybe, perhaps, some decrease in cognitive side effects.

In the meeting, Dr C tells me that radiotherapy of any kind has serious side effects, and particularly in Millie's case, because of the location of the tumour (it's not our fault, Guv – here we go again). Acute short-term side effects include fatigue, hair loss (actually this is permanent, I am told, on the areas the photons enter and damage healthy cells on their way to their tumour site), headaches requiring steroid treatment (in particular if there is some benign tumour left in the brain), and appetite loss. These short-term side effects occur irrespective of whether we go for photons (conventional radiotherapy) or protons (new and improved radiotherapy). Late side effects include a decline in Millie's endocrine functions relating to the pituitary, but these are already damaged, so not so relevant.

More relevant are the long-term side effects relating to loss of cognitive ability and second malignancies. And these are reduced by the use of protons. Given my objective as a parent is to ensure the best possible quality of life for Millie should she survive cancer, the decision for me turns on minimising those long-term side effects. Millie has enough to deal with without having to worry about loss of cognition and a second malignancy. I share my view with Dr C and she confirms that the type of tumour Millie has is not currently on the indications list (i.e. it does not yet qualify as a type of tumour for which proton beam therapy is made available through the NHS), but she feels it would be worth putting the case forward for consideration of NHS funding. It will take about three weeks to get validation. The recommendation put forward by Dr C goes to three independent panels, who would review Millie's case and then advise for or against funding. Unanimity is required. Sounds complicated; but I pretty much made up my mind there and then, funding or no funding, Millie is going to have proton beam, no matter what the cost (I have a figure of about £150,000 in mind, maybe more, all in).

We agree to meet again towards the end of the month and prior to Millie's third cycle of chemotherapy, this time at Dr C's clinic at University College London Hospital (UCLH), where radiology is located. At that point, we can review the decision on proton beam and go through the process of radiotherapy, which would include mask manufacture as well as a CT/MRI planning scan. It seems odd that the NHS would push for funding to such an extent, in particular for a condition that is currently not covered. Dr C knows more than she lets on, I'm sure. I'm just grateful that Millie will be considered for it.

I go back to Millie's room and update Vanessa on my conversation with Dr C. It's my turn to spend a couple of days and nights with Millie, so Vanessa leaves for East Sussex. To add insult to injury, Millie is now also on intravenous antibiotics for a possible infection in her right eye – something called preseptal cellulitis. For the unaccustomed, the orbital septum is a membrane of sorts, which is attached around the margin of the eye orbit. Preseptum means 'before the septum', so external to the orbit itself. They were worried at one point about a possible eye infection called orbital cellulitis, which is far more serious, with potentially life-threatening consequences and possible repercussions on vision, the optic nerve and the physiology of the eye itself. Thankfully, on this occasion, lady luck was on our side.

In any case, Millie's eye problem turns out to be a minor peripheral skin infection. Nothing serious, but it would have been nice not to have had it on top of cancer, the effects of Chemo Two and acute renal failure. It's more of the same for the next two days. Spending time in hospital is getting increasingly difficult. The days are long and it is hard to see Millie suffer so much. Frustration with doctors and nurses also often sets in. Everything happens slowly on an oncology ward, as if life itself were wrapped in a dreamy slumber.

We are finally discharged on the Sunday, but not before a platelet transfusion. Millie has now recovered from the eye infection, and although her blood count is declining, she is more herself and has regained some strength. She's been able to go to the playroom, where she played with a couple of the physiotherapists, throwing a ball back and forth by rolling it on the floor – some good signs of hand-eye coordination.

The bad news is that this time she has been prescribed a drug to boost white blood cells, called granulocyte-colony stimulating factor (G-CSF). This needs to be given sub-cutaneously (i.e. an injection in the leg) every day. Millie is clearly not happy about this. In itself, the injection is not a big deal, but when it comes on top of everything else, I can understand how she feels.

Reliable as always, Uncle Jonny comes to pick us up and we drive back home playing I Spy With My Little Eye. This time, we can spy a little further away and slightly smaller objects... Happiness is not an emotion I can often fathom nowadays, but as I hold Millie's hand on our way back home, I manage to find another type of comfort in the way her eyesight is continuing to improve. It's a small comfort, but it's perceptibly there.

# SO ON I FARED,
# IN THOUGHTFULNESS
# AND DREAD

*19) Day 61 – Tuesday 4th June*

Millie has been at home for over two weeks. Her blood count has gone down over this period, and she's needed another transfusion (chemotherapy seems to affect her platelets and red blood cells too). Her neutrophils and white blood cells have recovered more quickly this time, with the help of the G-CSF injections, and we were able to stop those after the first week (we were prescribed fourteen injections, one a day for a fortnight) as her white blood count was above 1.0 for two consecutive blood tests. She's recovering physically, but slowly.

Over the weekend, we even managed to go and fly some kites with Uncle Jonny at Mama's house. She was frail, slim, fragile, but still able to enjoy it, and with her vision slowly recovering every day, she was able to find her way to us up on the higher grounds and attempt to fly a kite, helped by her uncle.

It was almost a normal afternoon, after almost exactly two months of punishing regime, for her, for us, for our family. Two months has felt like an eternity – and the thought of two more cycles, one possible additional operation (it will actually turn out to be two more) and radiotherapy is difficult to grasp. These moments of normality are the ones I find the most difficult – because for one brief minute you forget the situation you are in. You are lulled into a false sense of security, unaware that the next big challenge is waiting, silent, arduous, testing every inch of stamina left in your body. But those challenges will come, and we have to keep our optimism in check at all times – it's the key to survival. Adopting a functional approach is the only way to be, but it requires effort and focus, and a detachment from our daughter as a parent. *One shot at a time.* Not always easy.

Millie is sleeping during the day – normally mid-morning and again after lunch, and we begin to notice disrupted sleep patterns at night. We often find the lights downstairs turned on in the morning, or in the middle of the night. This is probably a feature of the hydrocortisone she is taking but we are not certain at this stage, and the full effects of this particular drug have not completely kicked in yet.

Yesterday, Millie went up to London with Vanessa for her mid-treatment MRI scan. We had been told about this at the beginning of her treatment. After two cycles of chemotherapy, an MRI scan is undertaken to ascertain the degree to which the drugs are having an effect on the size of the tumour. Dr H expects the chemotherapy to have had an effect after the second cycle when it has unleashed its destructive powers on the cancerous cells. We expect the results back today.

We know the multidisciplinary team at GOSH meet every Tuesday morning, and they will all be looking at Millie's MRI scan in a pseudo-classroom environment, reviewing her progress and discussing the next steps. It's a tense morning for Vanessa and me. We know a call will come at any time to tell us whether or not chemotherapy is beginning to have an effect on the cancerous cells. It's possibly a defining moment in Millie's life. If the drugs have not been effective, we're in for some tough decisions – and it is likely that Millie will not survive the year. Sure, there's complete removal of the tumour, but at this stage, we don't know how effective that type of surgery will be, and we don't know what would happen afterwards. Possibly radiotherapy, but what would it mean for Millie's chances of survival?

The morning drags on. Lunchtime comes and still no call. Finally, at about 1pm, the phone rings and I pick it up. Dr H is away at a conference on children's brain tumours in Poland (I can't imagine the after-dinner entertainment would be much fun at an event like that, but then I suppose it's a job like any other). It's Dr M, who I also like. He's a good chap, with reflective eyes and tone, clearly intelligent and moderate in his approach. His tone is tentative and I can sense that he needs to deliver some uneasy news. It's the first time he's needed to get involved, as I normally talk to Dr H, so there is also possibly a degree of nervousness about approaching a difficult subject with a patient's father – especially the father of a seven-year-old with cancer. I know these guys do it day in and day out, but it can't be an easy task. I'm sure that although it's part of the job, empathy must kick in and they must feel a degree of emotional attachment to the people they are treating.

Dr M tells me that following the two courses of chemotherapy, the MRI scan shows a change in the tumour, with treatment-induced cysts resulting in a slight enlargement. This is not unusual but it takes me a few seconds to process. So, after two cycles of chemotherapy Millie's tumour has got *bigger* because of the cysts. After a few questions, this is what I understand: the tumour was a mixed mass of both benign and malignant stuff. Chemotherapy affects malignant cells by altering them such that they begin to die (it mostly acts on fast dividing cells and effectively stops them from reproducing). Dead cells are washed away (hmmm… not very scientific so far) and leave 'holes' in the tumour (especially in the kind of tumour Millie has, as the benign bits of her lump are unaffected by chemotherapy). When litres are pumped into the body during the intensive cycle, these holes fill with liquid and form cysts. The cysts and liquid inside of them increase the volume of the tumour.

Dr M tells me that the team feels this is not likely to improve with two further courses of chemotherapy. It will probably only aggravate the situation, and given the initial symptoms and possible pressure on optic nerves, they feel that an operation now, rather than at the end of the fourth cycle, is probably the best course of action. Millie's neurosurgeon Mr J happens to have a free slot tomorrow morning, so how are we set for coming up to GOSH later this afternoon for admission and for Millie to undergo her second craniotomy first thing?

We know it is not a question we are expected to say *no* to. Like a bad dream near dawn, all the memories of the first operation start flashing back: the conversation with the neurosurgeon on possible operative risks; the operation and waiting for it to finish; the worries relating to uncertainty of outcome; resus; the two or three days in the high-dependency unit; the tubes coming out of her; and the period of additional recovery she will need to get back to where she is at now (which ain't much). All of it comes flooding back, and also for Vanessa, judging by the look on her face.

After discussing non-options with Dr M, I am certain that the collective judgment of a team of specialists, who, ultimately, only have the best interest of their patient at heart, should be trusted in this instance. Besides, what's the alternative? Choice is an illusion in these circumstances. And Mr J will be operating. He's GOSH's lead neurosurgeon, and the one who pushed for the operation a couple of months ago, mobilising a full operating team to come and work on a Sunday, and who, by the looks of things, may well have saved Millie's eyesight as a result of that particular decision.

We tell Millie about the operation. She reacts to the news with the usual stoicism that has become her common currency for matters relating to her illness. She begins packing some of the things she wants for hospital and we start rallying the help we need to look after the other two. As both Vanessa and I will be going up to London for this, we pack for ourselves, taking a couple of days' worth of clothes and other essentials. Uncle Jonny drives us to Tunbridge Wells station and we make it to GOSH by mid-afternoon.

We meet with Dr M (Dr H will be back tomorrow morning from his conference) and Millie is formally admitted to GOSH: blood pressure taken, blood test done, bracelet with her name on it etc. I don't remember much of the day, but I do remember a conversation with Mr J (the lead neurosurgeon) about the operation and the risks associated with it. They are the same as the first operation – with one material difference. By now, Millie has regained probably 50% of her sight, and one of the main risks of the operation is total loss of vision (complete blindness). I ask Mr J if he is able to quantify that for us, and he says he doesn't like to do that as every case is different. I push him for an answer and he confirms one in five. That's high, and so much more difficult to cope with than the first time. The objective of the last operation was to preserve the little vision Millie had left. In many ways, the risk of total loss of vision then was a non-risk, because she had so little to lose. But now, with the vision coming back, it seems such an unfair risk for her to have, given her illness and all the possible outcomes. The concern is, of course, compounded by the fact that we're not going to know until the operation is finished, so we have plenty of time between now and then to do some serious worrying.

Mr J goes on to explain that, while still a craniotomy, this operation is going to be different to the first one Millie had. They will use the same incision line (that's good, only one scar), but will access the tumour site from above this time, rather than from the front, so we should expect less swelling of the eyes. In many ways, he explains, this will be an easier operation than the first. Not because it is less risky or less complex (it isn't), but because the objective of it is better defined: to remove as much of the tumour as possible. The first operation was a rescue mission in the dark. He didn't know what he was going to find, and what exactly he could do to debulk and relieve pressure on the optic nerve. This time, there's a plan, and the aim is clearer. What he doesn't know is *how much* of the tumour he will be able to remove. He will be chipping away at it a tiny fraction at a time, but he's uncertain of the consistency, and the degree to which healthy tissue around it is compromised or attached to the tumour so that removing its margins makes it more difficult without the risk of damaging healthy brain matter (optic nerves, pituitary and hypothalamus being the principal structures to avoid). He also says that the tumour is so big it has displaced the hypothalamus such that he doesn't know how it will affect the operation. Will the hypothalamus have moved in such a way to block access to the tumour and will damage to healthy brain tissue be inevitable, however much care is taken in avoiding that?

I fall asleep dreading tomorrow, not before arguing with one of the nurses who doesn't want to let both Vanessa and me stay the night. We stay the night in the end, but it's a fight I could have done without.

Of course I am apprehensive about the operation, but perhaps less so than the first time in terms of the risks associated with general anaesthesia, stroke etc. Millie coped well the first time, so we're not expecting this one to be different. Of course, I feel for my daughter who is the one who has to go through it. Holding her hand and caring for her is the easy bit. What worries me the most is the risk to her eyesight. This time the risk is not partial impairment or worsening of it – the risk is total loss. It's all or nothing.

I know I must stay positive. I know I must stay focused for Millie. I know this is the right thing to do. And so on I must fare, in thoughtfulness and dread. There is no choice in this particular game of life. We *have to* roll the dice and hope the numbers come out right.

## 20) Day 62 – Wednesday 5th June

The day of the second craniotomy is exactly two months to the day Millie started complaining of fuzziness in her eye, and therefore two months exactly since diagnosis of her brain tumour. Since then, she has had one craniotomy and two full cycles of chemotherapy. She has regained some of her vision and lost all of her hair. She has one more craniotomy to go (actually, it will turn out to be two more – but we don't know that at this stage) and two cycles of chemotherapy (which will end up being easier on Millie and significantly shorter than the first two, but we don't know that either).

We sign the consent form, which goes through the risks we had already covered in our conversation with the neurosurgeon. Under 'statement of health professional', the intended benefit of the operation is listed as 'Improve prognosis'. The risks are the ones we know, but the tangible nature of pen and paper casts them firmly into reality. They include: infection, bleeding, CSF leak, hypothalamic dysfunctions and endocrine disturbance, visual loss (there, thrown haphazardly and matter-of-factly among the rest), residual tumour (not sure that's a risk, the consequence of there being some residual is the risk), end of life, stroke, seizure and a last one I can't quite read – though I figure it can't be as bad as visual loss or end of life, so I live with the ignorance of it.

I don't know if it's part of the strenuous, taxing routine we have been subjected to or our experience of a previous similar operation and two aggressive sessions of chemotherapy, but somehow the risk of vision loss plays on my mind more than loss of life. I think it's because subconsciously I know one risk is significantly greater than the other. Loss of life relates to the operation or complications as a result of it, during or after. This risk is minimal and probably less than before given she had a similar operation two months ago and coped well. Vision loss is one in five.

We are eventually called to theatre after a mix-up with nil by mouth timings, which annoyed me more than anything else so far, because it could have risked another person being operated on first, therefore using a couple of hours' worth of Mr J's concentration, and I was keen for *all* his concentration to be used to remove Millie's tumour. The nil by mouth incident was not the first time basic maths had come in the way of a bad decision (I learned that nurses are very caring people, but not particularly gifted when it comes to simple arithmetic).

Millie chooses to walk alongside Vanessa and me – accompanied by the nurse on duty. It seems a long way to the operating theatre. I look down on her and know the next couple of weeks are going to be hard. Hard for her, hard for us. She is going to have to go through it all again and she is being so brave. She looks worried but puts on a brave face, for our sakes probably. She really doesn't have to – especially at the age of seven. We tell her again that the worst thing is feeling rotten for a few days, but that after that she'll start feeling better. We take her comforter 'Wawa' with us and give specific instructions to the team downstairs that it should be given to her as soon as she wakes. They acquiesce, a little bewildered. Millie's main concern is pain and possible injections – we reassure her that they will put her to sleep through her wigglies (Hickman line) and she will not feel a thing. Like last time, Millie opts to sit on my lap while they inject the first dose of anaesthesia that will send her to sleep. She's afraid, but tries hard to fight it. She really shouldn't have to go through this.

It is during these difficult moments that clarity about my current purpose in life is at its sharpest: I am here for her and no one else. What matters most is her comfort and wellbeing, as the patient and sufferer. Nothing else matters, not my feelings, my wife's feelings, or anyone else's feelings. Millie is the bottom line. The buck stops there and I live for her, and only her, in these hours, minutes and seconds that tick by.

She falls asleep and I gently place her on the small bed upon which she will be taken into operating theatre. I kiss her forehead and go back up to the ward with Vanessa. We know we won't hear from Mr J for another seven to nine hours. We hope for steady hands and a bit of luck, as he chips away at Millie's tumour, deep in the innards of her brain.

Up on the ward we meet Millie's oncologist Dr H, back from his conference in Poland. He is his usual cheerful, jovial self. He takes us aside to go through the latest events. As well as the MRI scan, GOSH also took blood to test for Millie's tumour markers, and he thinks the results may be back by now. A tumour marker is a substance secreted by a specific tumour and found in the blood. Millie's secreting germ cell tumour type often secretes chemical substances into the blood called alpha-fetoprotein and beta-HCG. Both of those were elevated when Millie was tested during the initial days following diagnosis. The more secreting germ cells you have, the higher the tumour marker, so they are often used to monitor treatment. But they are not the be all and end all. It is often the case, apparently, that a tumour becomes visible on an MRI scan before it is detected by tumour markers. But they are still helpful in providing an indication of trend and progress, and whether or not chemotherapy is having an effect on malignant cells.

Dr H looks up the results on one of the ward's laptops, while we are at his side. "The results are back... Let's see... Hmmm... They are down to 2.82." He seems pleased but nowhere near as pleased as I think he ought to be when he says, "They are back down to normal level. I was kind of expecting that." I repeat his last sentence in my head. *Millie's tumour markers are back down to normal levels.* They had decreased a little after the first cycle of chemotherapy, but after this second cycle the drop has been dramatic. This is brilliant news, though as always in our situation, we need to keep optimism in check. Her serum beta-HCG has returned completely back to normal from a height of 267 to 2.82 (normal range being 0-4). This is not only brilliant but *significant* in its reach and potential implication. Although they won't admit it, I also think it nudges that five-year survival rate percentage up a little. It must do, if only statistically, given 65% is the percentage at the beginning of the treatment. It means the malignant cells that make up part of Millie's tumour have been very sensitive to chemotherapy. It means that whatever malignant cells there are left in her brain, they are not sufficient in number to produce a tumour marker higher than the normal range. It doesn't mean she's cured of cancer, of course. In many ways, one never is – or it would certainly feel that way in time. Nevertheless, this is a massively positive step in the right direction: the first element of good news relating specifically to her cancer that we had received in the last two months.

Millie has only been in theatre for an hour or so. We know there's approximately seven hours to go and at least four hours before we are likely to hear anything at all, so we go to our usual Pret a Manger near Russell Square tube station to grab a bite to eat and update everyone on the status of the operation: "No news, but she went in at approximately 10:30am. Oh, and there's a one in five chance she'll come out blind, but at this stage there's nothing we can do about it..."

We wait and wait and wait. Nine hours is a long time to wait for the outcome of the single most significant event of your life so far. How successful has the surgery been in removing all, most, some of the tumour, and can Millie still see? We go back to GOSH and assume our usual position just outside the ward, where we try and distract ourselves by watching a movie on my iPad (*Salmon fishing in the Yemen*. A favourite of mine, and I lose myself in the story, its humour and the brilliant acting for a couple of hours). Seven hours go by and we don't hear anything, then eight, still nothing. Finally, we get word that Millie is out of the operation and is in resus, and that Mr J should be up with us at any time.

Mr J finally comes through the ward's door and reassures us instantly. "It's gone very well – she's fine, and she can see." He tells us that while the operation was easier in the sense that he knew what he needed to do (i.e. remove the tumour), it was technically a very difficult operation. He tells us that he measures difficulty according to the stress he undergoes during these procedures, and by counting how many hours or days an operation has shortened his life by. Because of the stressful nature of their work, apparently many neurosurgeons don't make it past their first year of retirement. Mr J rides a motorbike, so I point out to him that statistically he might not make it to retirement age anyway (oh dear, I'm turning into my parents). "I would say this operation has shortened my life by six months – no joke," he replies. I'm not laughing.

Mr J goes on to tell us that he feels he has managed to remove the whole of the lump without any damage to surrounding tissues. After the news on the tumour markers, this is turning out to be a pretty good day. I look deep into Mr J's eyes and feel genuine love for this man I didn't even know existed until two months ago. How do you express gratitude commensurate with the degree of success that's been achieved? Not only was he the person that most likely saved Millie's eyesight (in time, it would return to almost normal, including her peripheral range – a very rare occurrence), but he also managed to take the entire tumour out in an area where it is difficult to do so (the brain) and therefore, potentially, improve the prognosis significantly.

Two days later, the post-operative MRI scan would confirm complete resection. In other words, no visible tumour left. He had managed to take everything out. What's more, he described the MRI scan as one to 'frame and put on a wall'. It was *that* good. The only short-term uncertainty left (there were still many long-term ones, including whether or not Millie would survive five years) was the result of the histopathology. They would analyse what they had taken out to measure how many malignant cells were still remaining. If there were some remaining, the presumption was that there were some still left inside of Millie's head. If none were found, then it would be assumed none would have been left in Millie – sounds logical.

The small tremors that have been threatening us all day have not grown into anything more sinister. There was no darkness at the end of it. Today was a good day and the day is at an end. All is quiet and all is calm. We go to resus and find Millie as we expect after an operation of this magnitude. The last two days were not easy; not easy for us and not easy on Millie who had to go through a nine-hour craniotomy – but they were worth it. We *know* we are in a better place as a result of our focus to be functional in our approach to this nightmare, our trust in the collective guidance and outstanding brilliance of the multidisciplinary team at GOSH and our determination to keep to the task at hand whenever we are asked to do so by them.

*21) Day 69 – Wednesday 12th June*

Millie came out of the high dependency ward about four days ago and we know the drill and most of the staff by now, having already spent ten days here a couple of months ago. There are observations, urine output measurements, various anti-sickness drugs and endocrine fumbling about with dosages. It's a slow recovery this time, and she has suffered from nausea for a few days. She is barely eating, and whatever she is eating (or drinking) comes back up regularly. We were about to be discharged on the Sunday when she developed a temperature. Given our experience after the first cycle of chemotherapy I decided it was safer to stay an extra night. We end up staying an extra five nights, during which her weight dropped to 17kg (i.e. she lost 20% of her body weight in five days – it would be like me losing two stone in just under a week). Once again the blood culture comes back negative.

In the end, the neurosurgeon feels it could be hypothalamic. This organ may well have been irritated or disturbed during the operation. The hypothalamus, amongst a myriad of things, is responsible for controlling body temperature. Put simply, the body keeps its core temperature constant by physiological adjustments controlled by the hypothalamus, where there are neurons sensitive to changes in skin and blood temperature. This may well have been what happened the first time we came out of GOSH and ended up in our local hospital, when Millie had a temperature but no associated infection. We are told the only thing for it is to wait. Although by this stage it is also likely that the lack of food has destabilised Millie to such a degree that she may have developed hypoglycaemia, which is worsening her condition and ability to keep food down, which in turn is worsening her hypoglycaemic state.

The level of excellence and care I admired so much when this all began is now beginning to grind. I get easily annoyed by the nurses, I am beginning to be more knowledgeable than they are about the specific medicines Millie is taking, and I am most definitely more efficient at administering the right doses at the right time. All of this upsets me, not because of some self-serving narcissistic inclination, but because getting it wrong makes Millie suffer all the more. My particular bug-bear is the way in which desmopressin is administered. Before each dose is due, the endocrine team requires a sodium reading, to cover their arses – figuratively speaking. If the sodium level is within the normal range, Millie is given a miniscule amount of the drug that stops her from drinking litres. Because things in an NHS hospital (outside of really critical situations or intensive care) never happen on time, the dose is always given late, which means Millie drinks more than she ought to until the medicine is actually given. This makes endocrine review the dose further and take more sodium level tests, and so on and so forth. I have it out with one of the endocrine registrars (I don't mean kissing) to explain that while I may not be an endocrine specialist (thankfully), I understand how to measure properly, and moving the goalposts on an ongoing basis is not the answer. If you want to see the effects of a causal variable (i.e. desmopressin), you have to manipulate that variable alone whilst keeping everything else constant. This is not what's happening here. In the end, I actually grow fond of the endocrine team looking after us, and in particular three of the doctors there – Vaida, Claire and Caroline, and Prof E, under whose care we still are, though sadly both Claire and Caroline have now moved on. They may have been a pain (in the genuine pursuit of doing their job), but at least they genuinely cared and listened, and sometimes, that's all us parents ask for.

I am due to meet Millie's oncologist radiologist, Dr C, for the second time later today to discuss the next stage of treatment for Millie. We have just been told by Millie's oncologist, Dr H, that we have been approved for proton beam therapy. This is *amazing* news, as it is the best and latest available treatment – and the NHS will be funding much of it. I was always clear that Millie was going to receive it, but being helped along by the NHS feels like a bonus. I know there is no such thing as government money, only tax payer's money, but I still think it's amazing that the only costs I have had to date are the train tickets from Tunbridge Wells to London and back, and the various toys I have bought for Millie over the last two months. This is set to continue: I will not pay for proton beam either.

The other comfort comes from the approval process itself. My take is that the NHS wouldn't consider committing funds of this magnitude for a single seven-year-old girl if it didn't believe there was a better-than-average chance for complete cure. Despite some criticisms it has received of late, the NHS is a commercial organisation, and I find it reassuring that it is betting on Millie to survive cancer – perhaps more reassuring than the oncologist's opinion on percentage survival rates. Part of me also feels there might be another hidden agenda that us lowly parents of patients are not privy to. Not a sinister one, just a different one to the seemingly altruistic one of offering a young girl with cancer, that's not on the list of pre-approvals, the chance to go and have proton beam abroad, courtesy of the NHS. This I would never find out, so it remains pure speculation to this day.

This time, I meet Dr C at University College London Hospital, with a team of people including M, who will later help in the organisation of the trip to the US. Ah yes, proton beam facilities do not exist in the UK, so we will have to go to one of two centres associated with GOSH: Jacksonville (Florida) or Oklahoma City (Oklahoma). We don't know which at this stage, and won't find out until about a month before we are due to go. According to Dr C, this won't be until late August, by which time Millie will have finished two more courses of chemotherapy and her blood count will have recovered enough for her to be able to fly.

Proton beam is quite topical at the moment, and it is around this time (actually August rather than June) that the UK government announces its commitment of £250m to build the first two proton beam facilities in the UK, in Manchester and London, to be completed by 2018. It will no doubt save lives and save costs (no more funded trips to the US), so there will be more to spend on research and cures – so vitally required in order to save the lives of future children in need of treatment.

I go back to East Sussex from UCLH and Vanessa comes up to London to take Millie home. It's time to take her out of hospital and care for her at home. At 17kg she is a shade of her former self, but a shade we can still see.

# THE ODOUR WHICH
# INFLAMES US WITH DESIRE
# TO FEED AND DRINK

*22) Day 78 – Friday 21st June*

After spending pretty much all the first three days throwing up, Millie is beginning to regain her appetite and also keeping food down. We were a little perplexed at GOSH's advice to start with a few mouthfuls of Lucozade to get blood sugar levels up. Vanessa, who is a qualified nutritionist and passionate about it, has gone back to basics the old-fashioned way. She started the first few days with homemade chicken stock to restore the lining of Millie's gut.

Millie's weight is beginning to go up. This is a relief at first, but then it starts becoming a little concerning. What started as a healthy appetite at mealtimes is slowly becoming an uncontrollable hunger 24/7. Food starts to go missing, and we notice that Millie's night-time activities include eating (mostly breadsticks, fruit bars, crisps, that sort of thing). Her stomach is expanding a little every day and her face is beginning to look a little too round and swollen for comfort.

We'd heard that excess hydrocortisone could be the cause; or hypercortisolism, being the range of conditions characterised by an excess of circulating corticosteroids. A variant of it is known as Cushing's syndrome, and may arise from the adrenal cortex, e.g. because of an adrenal tumour, or may be secondary to overproduction of pituitary adrenocorticotrophic hormone (ACTH). The most common cause of hypercortisolism is, however, steroid therapy. And we think that is what's causing the swelling and rapid weight gain. The perplexing element is her change in behaviour and the obsession with food and eating all of a sudden. Millie has been on steroids since 5th April of this year and on hydrocortisone since mid April. So why the change? We don't know, GOSH doesn't know and the endocrine team is even suggesting it may be a result of the latest operation and possible damage to the hypothalamus, which is also involved in regulating hunger. Is there anything the hypothalamus doesn't control? Does it control my urge to scream at the top of my voice whenever we encounter additional trials that come on top of already colossal challenges? Perhaps.

The neurosurgeon, Mr J, does *not* believe the hypothalamus was damaged during the operation. He suggests it may be related to chemotherapy. Oncology feels it must be something to do with Endocrinology. They, in turn, think it might be neurosurgery. It's beginning to feel like builders blaming each other's workmanship. We arrange to meet with the consultant endocrinologist when we are next at GOSH for Millie's third cycle of chemotherapy. This was meant to start in four days' time, but given the slow recovery from the second operation we agree to review how she feels the day before the third cycle is due to start and postpone by a week if necessary. There is always a fine balance between killing cancer cells and killing the patient when administering chemotherapy. I'm sure a week won't make much of a difference, and so far we've been extremely compliant with GOSH's last-minute requests. We feel it would be better if Millie was allowed an additional week to recuperate (and probably put on more weight, unfortunately, as if irreversibly drawn to the pleasant smelling tree, where goodly fruitage hangs).

*23) Day 81 – Monday 24th June*

We travel up to London to meet with our oncologist Dr H to review Millie's progress and see if she is fit to start her third cycle of chemotherapy tomorrow or if we can wait one week and start it the following Tuesday. She is not doing badly: she is slow and generally weak, of course, but overall can generally keep up, although she needs carrying around now and again. Her eyesight is improving perceptively every day, which is beyond what we had hoped (and it will, by the way, continue to get better over the coming months).

Today is a huge day as far as Millie and her prognosis is concerned. This is because we gain the knowledge of three material results linked to the operation and chemotherapy, though the third will be the consequence of the other two.

- The first is this, and it is such a game changer that I will reproduce what has been written in the letter from Dr H following the operation and the histopathology, the results from the analysis of the lump that was removed, and which have now come back. My emphasis is in the quote below: 'Millie underwent a craniotomy by Mr J, her neurosurgeon, on 5th June and a *complete macroscopic resection* of her tumour was obtained, as confirmed by a postoperative MRI scan of her brain and reviewed by the neuro-oncology MDT'. I believe MDT stands for mechanical diagnosis and therapy. To an extent, we already knew this as we were told as much after the operation, but to see it in writing, with the benefit of distance from the emotional intensity of the operation, gives me a sense of accomplishment that I hadn't experienced before.

• The second result is another game changer. And so, here are the words I have read and savoured over and over again (my emphasis in italics): 'The histopathology of this (resection) showed tumour consistent with a germ cell tumour but with mature teratomatous elements *dominating* with only a *few* cells with somewhat *doubtful* staining for beta-HCG, and overall it was felt that there were *no malignant viable elements* in the residual'. This is an incredible sentence. Not only is *all* of the tumour out, but what was taken out was mostly mature teratoma, the most likely benign element, with only a *few* cells with *somewhat* doubtful staining for beta-HCG (i.e. the few cells that were found to be malignant were most probably in their dying phase). This means by implication that anything left inside of Millie at the mircoscopic, cellular level must also mirror the histopathological characteristics of what was taken out. Nothing is visible to the naked eye and tumour markers are now normal.

When you've numbed your emotions deliberately for a few months it is difficult to feel elation (and it would probably be wrong to do so in any case), but this is the best news we have had to date about Millie's condition. It certainly improves her prognosis, though Dr H wouldn't move on that one – still 65% – either he does not understand statistics, or he is keen to continue to manage expectations.'

- The third is a consequence of the first and second piece of news. We hear what are perhaps the two most significant words whilst in the process of curing cancer: *complete remission*. Millie is now, clinically at least, in complete remission, as the cancer can't be visually detected on scans or in blood tests. In other words, there is nothing left *that can be detected by blood tests or scans*. That's not to say Millie is cured – far from it, but it's a good place to be. While we will still follow protocol and finish two more cycles of chemotherapy, and then radiotherapy in the form of proton beam, the chemotherapy administered may well be weaker as a result and therefore easier on Millie, though this is yet to be confirmed. This is also good news because of Millie's acute kidney failure the last time around (and another reason why future chemo cycles may be altered in some way). Here, the latest GFR (kidney function test) has shown signs of recovery (phewww!), and following discussion with the intracranial germ cell tumour working group in Europe (critical life-saving decisions at GOSH are not made by single consultants, thankfully) they are going to switch cisplatin (the likely culprit of kidney failure) with carboplatin and keep the other two drugs (etoposide and ifosfamide). The practical implications of this will mean a more tolerable chemotherapy, with less fluid involved, and administered over three days rather than five. This also means less time spent afterwards to rebalance Millie from an endocrinological perspective.

The road is still long, the outcome uncertain, but in three defining events, pain is *slowly* turning into solace.

Following protocol is important in the context of curing cancer. Most remission statistics are based on this or that protocol, relating to this or that trial, this or that empirical study, or, just plainly, this or that empirical evidence. Millie is following PEI protocol as discussed earlier in this diary. As a result of recent encouraging results, Millie will now be following CarboPEI, which is used for a type of tumour called a germinoma (it is also easier on the kidneys, the most likely reason for the switch). My understanding is that CarboPEI is actually the protocol used in the US for the cancer Millie has. Different countries adopt slightly different protocols according to, I suspect, a variety of criteria such as interpretation of clinical trial, empirical evidence of previous treatments, costs vs. benefits and so on and so forth.

So while we are changing her treatment, we are still following protocol. This is very important. Millie is on an overall protocol that directs her broader cure with a multimodality of treatment, which is applied to children with her condition. Ignoring emergency surgery at the very beginning, this includes chemotherapy to reduce the tumorous mass, surgery to take out whatever is left and radiotherapy to minimise the chances of recurrence.

Millie's third cycle of chemotherapy comes and goes without us noticing much. She was admitted on the Monday. Vanessa took her in and spent the first two nights – although the second night ended up being the last night. By the time I come up to London on day three, the last drug is due to be administered later in the afternoon, and there's just enough time to go and see Millie's endocrinologist, Prof E to get Millie formally registered with him at his clinic next door.

This is bizarrely located within the buildings of the Royal London Homeopathic Hospital. I don't know if they still practice homeopathy there, I certainly hope they don't. They measure and weigh Millie with precision. She weighs 21.2kg and is on the twenty-fifth centile for her age, and stands at 115.8cm – the ninth centile.

It is clear she is small for her age, and Prof E had already indicated that she was likely to require growth hormones. But this would not start before the treatment for her tumour was finished, so at some point towards the end of the year, once proton beam was over. We talk about our concern over her weight, as she is gaining a kilo a week at the moment. We also get confirmation of the need to establish, over time, whether she is ACTH deficient (ACTH being adrenocorticotropic hormone, which stimulates the adrenals to produce cortisol), due to the disease process (i.e. her tumour damaging the pituitary). Alternatively, whether the adrenal axis is suppressed secondary to exogenous (external) steroids. This relates to the steroids given to Millie, and specifically the high dose of dexamethasone which was given to her right at the beginning to lower the swelling, but which, unfortunately, has suppressed the production of ACTH.

After some bartering (and my soliloquy on the detriment of hydrocortisone), Prof E agrees to lower the dose further from 10mg to 7.5mg. This is still just over replacement dose, but Prof E feels it would not be prudent to reduce it further prior to reviewing her cortisol profile (for which we will be admitted over the course of the next couple of weeks). Cortisol profiling means coming in overnight and measuring the level of cortisol in Millie's system, to establish the lowest possible dose she can be placed on, until we ascertain whether her pituitary is still capable of producing ACTH. We won't be able to do that until the end of proton beam therapy, as even this type of radiation could have a detrimental effect on the functioning of the pituitary gland. Generally nothing medical, or specifically endocrinological, happens quickly, so I accept this 'win' of a reduction in dose for the time being. We also agree to meet again in four months to start the process of growth hormone therapy, as Millie will no doubt need it. If she doesn't already, then she certainly will by the time protons have irreparably damaged the cells in her pituitary.

We go back to GOSH, where Millie is administered her last dose for this cycle. Compared to the previous two cycles of chemotherapy, this has been a breeze, though I can talk... I'm not the one who is being injected with venom. And she is well enough to go home. Uncle Jonny comes over to help, but this time, Millie is well enough for us to be able to take the train. I don't want to give readers a sense that she is *well* at this point. Compared to a healthy child, her energy level, concentration level and ability to be self-sufficient is running at about 30% of normal. But she is well *enough* to take the train with us, though I still have to carry her for much of the way as she can only walk a few hundred yards before becoming too tired to continue.

We arrive home and Millie asks for food. Not even chemotherapy has managed to diminish her sensitivities to the odour which inflames her desire to feed and drink. And at seven, with a brain tumour and hormonally imbalanced, temperance is not a virtue she is allowed to possess.

# A LITTLE GLIMPSE OF SKY
## WAS SEEN ABOVE

*25) Day 104 – Wednesday 17th July*

Ellie and Luca have now finished summer term at school, so caring for Millie requires a little more logistical focus. Luckily, the school my children attend organises summer courses, which start next week. Meanwhile, Millie had her cortisol profile test yesterday. Nothing too involved – basically blood tests taken periodically, on the dose of hydrocortisone Millie is on, to find out if the dose of replacement steroid is too much or too little. It is important for people on replacement steroids that the dose is enough to ensure they remain well, but equally important to ensure the dose is not excessive. We think it is, but we happen to be wrong on this one. Actually, it's not that we doubt the accuracy of dosage, more that we believe that the hydrocortisone, even in the small quantities Millie is taking, is adversely affecting her (wrong again). We find out the results of this analysis later today. It is also today that I will get confirmation of where we will end up for Millie's proton beam therapy. Currently, GOSH has a relationship with two centres: one in Jacksonville, Florida, and one in Oklahoma City, Oklahoma. A cursory look at both and their surrounding facilities quickly makes up our minds that we prefer Jacksonville, but ultimately, this is about curing Millie of cancer so we are not particularly fussed about where we end up. Just not Oklahoma City, pleeeease!

The oncology radiologist, Dr C, confirms that Millie has been accepted to the Oklahoma City facility... Hey ho! Prior to today I had read extensively about proton beam and, to a degree, Dr C's summary in clinic today corroborates the knowledge I have gained through, mostly, Google. So that's reassuring.

- Proton Beam therapy involves shooting protons as a way of irradiating the tumour/tumour bed, rather than photons, as in conventional radiotherapy (I will cover proton beam in detail in Part III of this diary). Because of the physics involved, protons release most of their energy *in situ* (where the tumour is/was) and effectively die out there. So there is a small entry dose and no exit dose. This is different with photons, as these enter, go through healthy tissues (damage them – bad), go through the tumour site (damage that – good) and then carry on their merry way out of the body (or head in this case, and damage those tissues too – bad).

- As a result of less healthy tissue being affected, Proton Beam radiotherapy reduces latent (or long-term) side effects; and the one that worries us the most – loss of cognitive ability ("with conventional radiotherapy if she were a grade A student, she'll go from a grade A to a grade C." Right. Is that in maths, physics or history of art?).

- Apparently, they are significantly more brutal in the US when going through consent and side effects. Dr C warns us to be aware of that and not to worry about it too much.

She tells me this at least three times on three or four different occasions. Okay, I get it.

- A mask will be made to fit Millie's head, which will be used when administering treatment. Depending on whether or not Millie can stay absolutely still, she may have to go under general anaesthesia every day whilst undergoing proton beam therapy. Let's hope she can lie still…

- And that's every day for six weeks – she will need thirty sessions in total, though they won't be longer than thirty minutes each and most of that will be spent aligning her body and head in the right position.

M, the admin assistant, then gives me a summary of what is likely to happen. Given where Millie is at treatment-wise, we are looking at mid-August to fly out to Oklahoma. The NHS will cover economy flights for Millie and two carers ('fare' enough…) and basic-but-comfortable accommodation, as well as one hire car. Flights won't be booked until Millie has recovered from her last cycle of chemotherapy and her last MRI scan needs to be clear. This will be sent to the centre in Oklahoma for final consent – this is called stealth MRI, for reasons I have not yet completely understood.

My head is beginning to spin slightly. The fact I will have to go 4,000 miles away for two months ("Expect to be there for longer than you expect," says Dr C), fills me with dread. I have never liked travelling far as I've never understood the point of going somewhere geographically different just because it's somewhere else. It's just as arbitrary as someone from that place coming to your neck of the woods because it's a different place than his residence. Granted, there are things like sunshine, sea and different cultures to learn about, but these days, whenever I go on holiday with my family, I spend most of my time on my own, seeking the shade. So I see even less of a point to it. In any case, that's holidays and this is different, so I'm going to have to think about organising our trip somehow or another. I'm already clear that we ought to go as a family (i.e. the five of us) but there is much to do before doing so becomes feasible.

On my way to East Sussex, I get the results back from Millie's cortisol profile test. It confirms that she needs the dose of hydrocortisone she is currently on – though they lower it to 6mg a day (from 7.5mg) after I go on about the detrimental effects, the lack of sleep, the hunger, the grumpiness etc.

Hydrocortisone has become yet another barrier against which we keep banging our heads, like a wall of flames that's kept in check, right in front of us, by a strong wind forming boundaries we are unable to reach or change.


*26) Day 105 – Thursday 18th July*


There are times when you really feel flat as a carer, and more specifically as a parent of a child with cancer. When problem compounds on to problem, especially at the beginning, it is difficult to see how you will ever escape the vortices that circle and entrap you in a nightmare world of serious illness, disease and the destructive cure of cancer. It isn't enough that our daughter has cancer, that her vision has been compromised, that she has had to endure two brain operations, three cycles of chemotherapy and one more to come, that she will have some of her brain cells destroyed forever by proton beam at some stage in the next two months, that she will require growth hormones every single day until she has finished growing and possibly beyond, that she cannot function without a daily dose of desmopressin without which her daily urine output and water intake is measured in gallons. And not to mention the obvious, that cancer may yet recur over the next five years. No. She also needs to take hydrocortisone, a drug that's making her want to eat, making her irritable, making her put on weight, and that will have worse consequences in the long term. That's if we're lucky. That's if this really is the hydrocortisone. She may well have a damaged hypothalamus. But GOSH doesn't seem particularly interested, which is disappointing, as we feel we might have to eventually start looking for alternatives elsewhere.

There are times when you feel that way. And you can't even begin to see the outlines of the day you hope for. Luckily, Millie is never too far away to remind us all why we try so hard.


27) *Day 119 – Thursday 1st August*


Millie's last cycle of chemotherapy started two days ago in Lion Ward. It was meant to begin last week, but her blood count had not recovered sufficiently. That they made us go all the way to GOSH, knowing the blood count, only to be told to go back home, wasn't helpful. That they made us wait until the last minute before telling us she would start on the Monday of this week, having been the ones to postpone her last session, had the appearance of unnecessary cruelty spawned by bureaucratic inefficiency. While I have no doubt GOSH saved our daughter's life by applying excellence when it really mattered, much improvement can be had in the daily management, administration and handling of patients with cancer. I'd be more than happy to make suggestions, for free, if they ever ask me.

The neurosurgeon, Mr J, comes to see us. We were meant to go and see him in clinic, but Millie being here meant he came to us. He is pleased with her progress and even more so when I show him a little video on my iPhone of Millie throwing a ball against a wall at home and catching it – repeatedly, accurately and without dropping it once. This level of hand-eye coordination was just unimaginable a few weeks ago, and it has only been made possible by Mr J's desire to save her eyesight at the beginning of April. I love that man, and I have a deep desire to kiss and hug him every time I see him, but I know that would be inappropriate.

Millie is about to be given her last dose of the last poisonous chemical to be infused in her body (for now anyway, who knows what the long-term future holds). What started on Tuesday 16th April, in a world still surrounded with uncertainties (including whether or not Millie would live to see this through), is about to come to an end. The last drop goes in. It's done. I never thought it would feel this good. I look at her and see a promise of better things to come. She did it. *She* did it. Supported by an incredible team at GOSH, but she did it – let no one take that away from her. I feel a sense of pride which I'm sure no future exam results or first prizes or learning how to play the fucking piano or anything I could possibly imagine will ever come close to.

I look out of the window on to the internal courtyard of GOSH, the one I used to stare at so often while waiting for Millie to come out of her first two operations. I look up, and through the grey clouds of an overcast London sky, I catch a glimpse of blue.

# FEEL THE EDGE OF OTHER SWORD; AND THOU SHALT WEEP FOR THAT

*28) Day 127 – Friday 9th August*

My parents come to visit this week all the way from Italy. This is a big deal for them as my mother is in poor (but improving!) health and my father doesn't travel much these days. He prefers the tranquillity of the familiar to the hustle and bustle of travelling – a trait I have probably inherited. They have been here a few days and Millie is really enjoying their company. I can see she finds it soothing and I'm grateful to them for making the trip. She even plays catch with my father and is relishing the experience. These moments with Nonna and Nonno are an essential part of healing – they restore memories of better times and go a small way towards erasing those of past pain.

*29) Day 133 – Thursday 15th August*

For the first time since April, I meet up with a couple of friends for a game of golf. I was also meant to go up to London afterwards to meet up with Clara, another good mate. Unfortunately, this is the day Millie chooses to feel unwell (not her fault obviously, and I don't blame her), so I need to head back home instead. Millie had a lumbar puncture yesterday, a minor procedure under general anaesthesia, to ascertain, post chemotherapy, that cancer had not spread down her spine. This was purely routine. It hadn't spread when they last checked back in April, so was unlikely to have done so since, especially given the intensity of treatment received. The procedure itself involves a minor operation in Safari Ward (GOSH's outpatient ward). Millie is admitted, assessed and then waits her turn with four or five others, to go into the 'operating theatre'. This is just a regular room where she is given a mild anaesthetic and a small amount of lumbar fluid is extracted (about 5ml, they tell me). After she wakes up, they just wait for her to eat, drink, go to the loo and then it's time to go home.

What they don't tell you is that more often than not this disrupts the fluid balance/pressure in the brain (it's all connected) so patients end up feeling nauseous the following day. This is exactly what ends up happening. Not equipped with this knowledge, we take her to Pembury hospital, and the doctor there confirms the nature of her discomfort. It's hard enough worrying about cancer, without having further unnecessary uncertainties on top of it. Just have a checklist to give to parents after these types of procedures, so they know what to expect when they get home!

As we already suspected, the good news is that the analysis comes back negative. Still no spread – and tumour markers still normal. If the cancer had spread to her spinal cord, this would have reduced the remission percentage from 65% to 20%. Good thing we caught this early enough, out of pure serendipity.

Oklahoma is getting closer and I've put feelers out to see if anyone I know has any connection with someone there, or the US. As luck would have it, my good friend Dom, or rather his mum (bless his heart – thank you Dom!), has a friend in Oklahoma City, a lady called Linda. We connect and I like her instantly. She is helpful, compassionate and supportive (to me! A total stranger!). In the end, she makes a significant difference to how well we manage to integrate in Oklahoma City (but I mustn't get ahead of myself – all of that will come in Part III of this diary). We have also touched base with ProCure's own patient support manager, but so far, she has been reticent to do too much. I think she might have guessed what was to come…

One of the final checks made before confirmation of our flights to Oklahoma is a stealth MRI scan – so called because… huhhh… still no idea. Anyway, this Millie had yesterday. It's her fifth MRI scan since April of this year – so she's pretty used to it by now and knows how to lie still. The results will be sent to ProCure, the proton beam centre in Oklahoma, to begin the plan of irradiation for Millie when we get there. It's also used to make sure that nothing has grown back since the last operation, so we're all pretty nervous about it (God knows how we will feel about the check-up MRIs six months down the line and a year down the line – those that confirm whether she is still in remission or if a tumour is growing once more. We'll think about that then, no point wasting energy now).

I call the hospital and talk to R, a lady who was meant to be our key worker and single point of contact with GOSH, hence removing the complexity of the workings of a large NHS trust. She was comprehensibly useless in that role, and can't help me much on the phone now either, as she hasn't been to the meeting they had this morning (this after trying to bleep her about seven times, without being able to reach her once). As I am in London, I wonder if I might just go and see Dr M, the oncologist covering for Dr H, who is on holiday at the moment. Thankfully he has a free slot later this afternoon.

I begin to be slightly uneasy about the whole thing – having always subscribed to the theory that if there's nothing wrong, the tendency is for lower level staff to tell you things over the phone. R's reluctance, I feel, may be hiding some complications. My instincts were right. The scan reveals another lump, though Dr M and the team do not feel this is a new tumour. It is mid-way between the tumour site and the surface, in the track used to access/remove the tumour last time. It appears to have some form of blood supply feeding it (possibly a blood clot?), so they will ask ProCure for a final confirmation about what to do next.

The overall consensus would have been to leave it there and then re-scan in a couple of months to see if the body has reabsorbed it. However, time is a currency we do not have in the context of treating cancer. The most likely outcome will be a third craniotomy in the next week, before flying to Oklahoma (which is now likely to be delayed by a week or so). Later that day, I speak to the neurosurgeon Mr J, who is far more straight-talking than the oncologist covering for Dr H. You know, it helps us parents when people are straight-talking. We do not need protection, we need facts so we can deal and cope with them in the way we know how, and organise our lives accordingly. Mr J is also very reassuring with regards to the nature of this lump: "It's something related to the last operation, probably a blood clot, but nothing to worry about." Still, one can't help but worry. He confirms that in his experience, the proton beam centre will ask for the lump to be removed. This is really to remove the uncertainty as regards to its nature, the theory being that proton beam is a one-shot strategy. What we can't do is have it and *then* find out that actually, this lump wasn't a blood clot at all and that the 1% risk of this being a further tumour had crystallised, but we can't go back and irradiate that area too. Well, one could in theory, but not under the funding of the NHS second time around and, more critically, not without further damage to the brain as a result of a second dose of radiation.

I'm more than irritated by this latest piece of news, but I do what I do best – I contextualise. It's easy to blame doctors and neurosurgeons for these events, but ultimately, since 5th April of this year, the decisions that have been made on Millie's behalf by all involved have been spot on. They have saved her life (for now) and her eyesight (for sure). These minor blips happen in all walks of life – I guess they also happen when curing cancer.

We don't know when this third craniotomy will happen (the third in four months!) but it is likely to be soon (i.e. probably next week). We don't break the news to Millie yet. We'll tell her a day or so before. She's doing so well and we don't want to worry her for a full week before it needs to happen. I feel the edge of yet another sword about to open her head for a third time, and I feel for my daughter, who is going to have to go through it all again.

It is in these moments that a huge mental effort is required to extend the visual field to the long term – to when twelve or eighteen months have elapsed, when beauty and virtue will circle us once more. All this will eventually be nothing but a bad memory – a dream of night. I suppose we can't get there without a few tears and some pain.

# PURE AND MADE APT FOR MOUNTING TO THE STARS

The day of Millie's third craniotomy – GOSH confirmed last Friday that we were to come up yesterday to be admitted. We told Millie on Sunday, to allow her some time to think about what she wanted to pack. She wasn't best pleased this time around (and I can understand why), although it is testimony to the little fuss she made on all previous occasions that we noticed her justifiable grumbling this time around.

The operation itself should be less involved, and this was confirmed to us by one of the neurosurgeons the evening prior to the procedure. It would last anywhere between two to four hours, and no complications are expected. It is still a craniotomy, and even though we have now gone through two of these in the last four months, it is still an operation of considerable complexity.

Mr J meets us prior to taking Millie down to the operating theatre and tells us something he would never say had he not been supremely confident of the outcome: "I will see you later this morning, when I'll tell you that everything has gone

181

very well." Bless your heart, Mr J. This time, for some reason, we needed that reassurance. We needed to have more certainty with regards to the outcome prior to the event itself. And instinctively he knew that.

Usual stuff re: the operation – and it breaks my heart that it has become so normal for us, that I don't even feel the need to repeat in this diary what has gone before. We take Millie downstairs, where she is courage personified. This time, she chooses Mummy's lap rather than mine to fall asleep on. She closes her eyes and hugs Mummy tightly. Within seconds of the anaesthetic flowing into her veins she is fast asleep. See you later, angel of mine, after Mr J tells us that 'everything has gone very well'.

Vanessa and I go for a walk in the now familiar neighbourhood surrounding Russell Square. We walk to Tottenham Court Road and have a coffee in Planet Organic, where we take the opportunity to update friends and family, before making our way back to the hospital.

Three hours and twenty minutes after Millie went into theatre, Mr J comes to see us to tell us she is now in resus: "Everything has gone very well," he says… He also tells us that while we still need histopathological confirmation that what has been removed is nothing serious, he believes it is gelatinous residue (of a gelatine they use during this type of operation to promote clotting, or to prevent clotting, I can't remember which). By some freak occurrence, a little bit had gathered mid-way down the track used to access the tumour, lost some of its watery content, hardened, and blood cells had started gathering around it.

On the fourth day following her operation, Millie is well enough to be discharged, and the best I have seen her look so far. It is the first time I catch a glimpse of the old Millie – as she reveals this second beauty cancer and chemotherapy had so far kept concealed.

*32) Day 148 – Friday 30th August*

We are being discharged from GOSH today and there's always some waiting around when you are being discharged. I catch up on the papers (*The Times* on my iPad, more specifically). It includes an article about the record-breaking transfer of Gareth Bale from Tottenham to Real Madrid for a reported sum of £82m. While I have no beef with the man himself, it sickens me to the core that people whose only skill is keepy-uppy are paid in a week what the lead neurosurgeon at GOSH is probably paid in a year. Sure, they can fill a football stadium every week, full of supporters who are actually indirectly paying the salaries of all twenty-two players on the field, plus those on the bench and both managers. This despite the fact that these supporters are on 0.001% of the wages received by the people they idolise. It's redistribution of wealth on a massive scale, packaged as entertainment. Millie's lead neurosurgeon, on the other hand, only *saves children's lives* every day. I'm glad we live in a world that gets its priorities right...

While in the process of being discharged, we also get confirmation that after insisting for this particular operation, ProCure Centre in Oklahoma City now wants us there before 11th September. This means getting there the weekend of 7th September. Ouch – that's in eleven days' time, and Millie is still in hospital recovering from a third craniotomy! We still don't have accommodation, and we'll need to change the flights that had been booked for us by a well-known, internet-based travel company, who had heard about Millie through a dad from school and very kindly agreed to pick up the bill to fly us all the way there and back. Amazingly generous, and such a magnificent gesture from a company with whom I'd had no previous contact.

The radiology department at UCLH had not been spectacularly helpful in organising the administration for our trip, and neither had the ProCure Centre in Oklahoma, plus no school placements had been secured for my other two children, who were coming with us. Fuck, fuck, fuckety fuck. Some preparation had, of course, taken place (more on that later), but looming deadlines always have a knack for focusing the mind; much like cancer and the risk of losing someone.

Though we won't be losing Millie for now. It looks like we'll be staying with her for a little while longer, or rather, she will be staying with us. She won't be journeying to higher realms, not yet in any case, as we prepare to proceed to the final intensive phase of cancer cure: radiotherapy.

### 33) Epilogue to Purgatorio

On Sunday 8th September we leave for Oklahoma City. This second phase of treatment has now come to an end. Chemotherapy started on 16th April, following a first craniotomy. It finishes with a third craniotomy to allow Millie to continue on her way to some sort of recovery. As to whether this will be a full recovery, i.e. will she live beyond five years, we don't yet know. But we know more than we did prior to the start of this second phase of treatment, and there is certainly more tangible hope for a good outcome now than there was four months ago.

What characterised the first two weeks (back on 5th April, straight after diagnosis) was grief, uncertainty and fear. The dominant themes of this second phase have been different. We have had time to adjust to her condition and we are now fully aware of the significant illness that has befallen our daughter. We've had the opportunity to evaluate and process our thoughts and feelings about it. And, in the end, we have come to the realisation that they are not important. What's important is Millie – *her* thoughts and feelings and how we can help her so that she can adjust to her condition in the best possible way. What's important is our focus to remain functional and break large problems associated with curing Millie into manageable tasks. Part of compartmentalising treatment into three broad categories is to help us manage the process. It ensures we remain focused on what needs to be achieved month by month without being overwhelmed (as we would undoubtedly be) by the enormity of the overall objective. This spans the next five years and includes complexities and uncertainties that make it impossible for us to conceptualise a solution or a way out at this stage.

In all honesty it has not been easy, least of all for Millie, who is the one who has had to go through first-hand the demanding pace of aggressive cancer treatment, with all that it entails, including four cycles of hard-hitting chemotherapy and another gruelling nine-hour craniotomy (plus a third four-hour-long one thrown in for luck). It hasn't been easy to see Millie suffer as much as she did (and will continue to do in the foreseeable future), and to see her decline physically in the way that she has. It has required a gigantic shift in mind-set to ensure we continued to be functional in our approach to this challenging situation. Moreover, Millie is not our only daughter. Balancing life with a seven-year-old afflicted with cancer and ensuring you give enough to your other two children so they are not too affected, takes energy and planning.

To say we were not ready for this is an understatement on an astronomical scale. Nobody teaches you how to cope with life when your daughter is diagnosed with cancer, and when the initial treatment is as brutal and fast-paced as the one Millie has had to endure.

Luckily, we were not alone in navigating the difficult waters of cancer treatment. As you would expect, GOSH played a vital part in guiding us through it and in ensuring we felt a degree of control about our situation, when, let's be honest, there was none there. In this critical period, when the jaws of cancer and its cure, which can at first be more devastating, first tightened their grip on Millie and were pulling her forcibly down into the abyss, GOSH provided light, comfort and leadership. They jumped right in and rescued her from darkness – both figuratively and literally. And they bought us time and tangible reasons to hope.

Much was achieved during that time. We know that Millie is now in complete remission, so there are no traces of cancer left on her scans or blood analysis. This is not to say there are no cancerous cells left. There may well be, and this is the reason we are continuing with treatment, in particular with proton beam. And Millie can *see*. She can see well. She is improving every day. She spotted a plane in the sky the other day, and can read small print. It's not perfect, but we would have taken this in a heartbeat if it had been given to us the day after her first operation.

Much has been achieved, much still needs to be done, many uncertainties remain. The most significant impact of Millie's cancer, now that she has regained full functional vision, will be at the endocrine level. She will require growth hormones and daily drugs to regulate some of the functions that the pituitary gland is no longer able to perform. One of those drugs is hydrocortisone – the most damaging one from a side-effect perspective. Millie looks very different as a result of this drug, too. She has put on a lot of weight in the last month, and is continuing to do so. And hydrocortisone may not be the culprit. The endocrine team suggests it may be damage to the hypothalamus rather than hydrocortisone, which is also irreversible.

When you are left with time to reflect (and that's pretty much all you can do when evenings descend on a paediatrics' oncology ward, and you are left alone in the dark), your thoughts turn inevitably to the future and to how this (if Millie lives through it) will impact on her life, her work and on the relationships she may or may not be able to have as a result of it. The lesson I have learnt in the last four months is that this is not the right way to look at it. We have to look at Millie as she is now, not as a collection of future limitations, according to *our* expectations, but as an opportunity for improvement, according to *her* potential. It is only by doing so that we will make her apt for mounting to the stars. And proton beam will help us get there. Oklahoma, here we come!

# III

## PARADISO
### *(HEAVEN)*

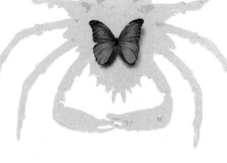

"Ma già volgeva il mio disio e 'l velle,
sì come rota ch'igualmente è mossa,
l'amor che move il sole e l'altre stelle."

*"But yet the will roll'd onward, like a wheel*
*In even motion, by the Love impell'd,*
*That moves the sun in Heaven and all the stars."*

Dante Alighieri, The Divine Comedy
*Paradiso – Canto XXXIII, lines 133-135*

"Her treatment's done. This course is run and we are on
our way."
*31) Day 211 – Friday 1ˢᵗ November*

# SO SAID, SHE TURNED
# TOWARD THE HEAVEN
# HER FACE

*1) Day 151 – Monday 2nd September*

GOSH confirmed Millie was due to be treated by the ProCure Proton Beam Therapy Centre in Oklahoma back in July. Now that we have clarity on our departure date, we also envisage having to stay there until at least the beginning of November. We will spend the first two weeks planning for treatment and then Millie will undergo thirty sessions of radiation therapy – one a day for six weeks, with week-ends off. So that's a further six weeks. Two months in total, maybe more. This requires planning, both for how we will spend our time in Oklahoma but also for the place we will be leaving behind for a couple of months.

The moving timeline of when we were due to start proton beam therapy has been unhelpful in planning for Oklahoma. The start was always going to depend on Millie and her recovery time through two further cycles of chemotherapy and, though we didn't know it, a third craniotomy. So, in a sense, the nature of the treatment makes it more difficult for us to plan. At the same time, we are also clear that we want to experience this as a family (i.e. the five of us) because we feel that the event is significant enough to warrant all of us being part of it. We want to make sure that our other two children don't feel left out, but perhaps more importantly because we are certain that Millie will benefit from all of us being there with her in Oklahoma City for the best part of two months.

We have to think about schooling, of course. Ellie and Luca are due to start term in a couple of days and we don't particularly want them idle for two months in Oklahoma (for our own sanity if nothing else). Their school in the UK has been very supportive about us taking them out until the beginning of November. Supporting my colleagues and covering for my role was going to be challenging, and also frustrating. But, of course, these are unimportant details in the context of curing Millie of cancer. To a degree, given the linear nature of time, I know Oklahoma will come and go. I know November will inevitably arrive and we will be back in the UK to reintegrate into some sort of normality. But it doesn't mean we can't make the most out of our time in the US – for all of our sakes.

I'd be lying if I didn't say I also feel a degree of apprehension about taking my family away for two months to the US, to a place I've never been before, and not a holiday destination. I have little awareness of where we would be staying (no accommodation had yet been confirmed) or what Vanessa and I would do there with three children. I'd heard of Oklahoma as a state, of course, and the City itself. I had a vague recollection of a musical by that name, and one of the least original jokes of the more moronic members of my immediate circle of acquaintances was to break into the headline song whenever I mentioned Oklahoma City. I also recalled the Oklahoma bombing back in the mid-1990s, oh yeah, and tornados. My initial search turns inevitably to Google, and Wikipedia in particular. This is broadly what I find:

- Oklahoma City is the capital of the US state of Oklahoma and its largest city. It is twenty-ninth among United States cities in population – consisting of more than 1.2 million people; and is the eighth largest city in the United States by land area.
- It features one of the largest livestock markets in the world. Oil, natural gas, petroleum products and related industries are the largest sector of the local economy.
- The city lies in between three other large cities: Dallas (Texas), Wichita (Kansas) and Tulsa (Oklahoma).
- Since weather records have been kept, Oklahoma City has been struck by nine strong tornadoes, eight F/EF4s and one F5 (Fs being tornado strengths). On 3rd May 1999, parts of southern Oklahoma City and nearby communities suffered one of the most powerful tornadoes on record, registering as an F5. On 20th May 2013 (i.e. this year!), southern Oklahoma City, Moore, and other surrounding areas and suburbs were struck by another devastating EF5 tornado.

Right, so it's not huge, but large in terms of spread. It's Midwest America, and it's cowboy and tornado country. A quick scan of Google Maps and Google Earth reveals a place that reminds me of Phoenix, Arizona, where I'd been a few times for work-related reasons, but greener and not as big. As my colleague Anna takes pleasure in letting me know, the nineteenth most popular tourist attraction in Oklahoma City is a pigeon rehabilitation centre.

Like gazing directly at the sun, I am unable to sustain my focus for long enough to make out what lies ahead with any degree of clarity or acuity. Time to let go.

During the last five months, I've sent regular updates to all friends, acquaintances and people I'd met along the way as a result of Millie's treatment. These updates are about Millie, the progression of her illness, her chemotherapy cycles and various operations (I shared the first one I wrote in Day 28 of Inferno). The last one I sent made reference to Oklahoma, and made enquiries as to whether anybody knew of anyone, that might know of anyone, who might know of somebody, who lived anywhere near it – you get the gist. As luck would have it, my good friend Dom replied that he did. I have known Dom since my first month of living in London post university. He is a dear friend and I spent much time with him back then. Life took over and in the past eight years, with three children in tow, it's been much more difficult to spend quality face time with friends, and so it was with Dom. We had kept in touch nonetheless. It turns out one of his mother's good friends was living in Oklahoma City. Wow, wouldn't you know it!

A couple of emails later, I am speaking with Dom's mother's friend. Her name is Linda, she has a thing for Macleans Fresh Mint Toothpaste, and sounds helpful straight away. Not for the first time in the last five months, I am grateful for the generosity and kindness of strangers. She can definitely help, she says, and would start reaching out to various people in Oklahoma who should be able to assist in finding us suitable accommodation. At this point ProCure had done little in terms of providing accommodation options, and I was getting anxious at the lack of choice. So far, there were two properties, quite far out, but close to ProCure.

I decided the best approach was to apply the process I see happening day in and day out as part of my job. I'm finance director for the only central-London-based relocation company, and we help big corporations relocate their assignees to London. Time to practice what I preach. We would go to a hotel for two weeks (Oklahoma is not spoilt for choice on that front – or at least not where we want the hotels to be – most tend to be located, quite rightly, near the business district), and then hopefully Linda and her contacts, including her sister Paula, who works in real estate (this is getting better and better!) would comb the market and find an option for us to rent for a couple of months.

A couple of days later, Linda suggests that her friend Mary might be able to rent her house to us. Mary had been involved as a carer for someone with cancer at some point in her life and was keen to help. Amazing. I didn't want to be too pushy, so we would continue pursuing all options. I'm beginning to feel better about the whole thing, but we're nowhere near where I would like to be. One of the most difficult exercises in extrapolation is choosing a house remotely, 4,000 miles away in a place you've never been before.

Meanwhile, Ellie and Luca start school in the UK today (we decided to let them go for the next three days before leaving for the US), so it's a good opportunity to update the other mums and dads on Millie. Vanessa has resumed school run duty by now, though it took a while before she felt able to do it – and I can understand why. I had already chatted with the headmaster, who had given me support for full flexibility with regards to taking Ellie and Luca out for two months. Of course, now that they were coming with us to Oklahoma, I wanted to make sure this turned into a learning experience by enrolling them in a local US school. So far I had got an extremely positive reply from one. It had been recommended to me by the lady whose house we would eventually rent for the duration of our stay. The response from them was immediate, heartfelt and supportive. The only obstacle was that they did not have a place for my son, and I was keen to avoid duplicating school runs, particularly as the primary purpose of our visit was to focus on Millie and her treatment. We had a couple of nursery options for him, but they were not ideal.

In one of our many conversations, Linda also suggests I look at Casady School as a possible option, and indicates that she could speak to someone to help things along. I look up Casady and it seems great. I write an email to the director of admission, and after a couple of chases I receive a one-liner confirming that Casady would have a place for both my children (they would end up taking Millie every morning too – but more on that later). Brilliant!

Linda, Mary and Paula turn out to be central to how well we ended up settling into Oklahoma City and how comfortably we would spend our two months there as a family. They epitomised the generosity of spirit that still exists amongst human beings today. In that sense, Millie's tumour was a gift – it brought us kindness, compassion, care, consideration and warm-heartedness of the most unselfish type.

Like spots on the moon, we go through our busy lives rarely noticing these human qualities, and I am grateful that my family and I have experienced them in such formidable fashion. They have changed me to be a better person as a result.


*3) Day 157 – Sunday 8th September: am*


Millie is recovering well from the last operation, though she is still weak and has a couple of naps a day. She can't walk further than a few hundred yards without her legs getting tired. She has now put on some ten kilograms (nearly two stone) since her lowest point a few days after her second operation towards the beginning of June. This is at least a stone overweight, which isn't helping with the difficulty in walking. A stone is around a third of her previous body weight, so it would be the same as me putting on three and half stone over a couple of months.

To be fair, Millie has spent much of the last five months horizontally. Certainly, while she was in hospital at the beginning, she was far too frail and blind to do anything other than listen to her iTouch and lie on her bed. The chemotherapy cycles were pitiless in their capacity for exhaustion. Within a day of being injected with cytotoxic drugs, Millie would spend much of her time in a state of semi-awareness of her surroundings, preferring to withdraw from day-to-day interactions with people and objects. When she was at home, it was much the same. There certainly hasn't been any running or skipping, though she tested a few things out to see if she could still do them, like scooting and hula-hooping. Scooting was an achievement in itself because of the balance required and the fact that she could see where she was going. Hula-hooping and ball catching was a favourite – but again, five minutes of any physical activity and that was that. We tried hard not to be too expectant of Millie. We knew rehabilitation from this devastating cure was going to be measured in months (or maybe years…) rather than weeks, and we knew that the starting point – the base level from which to measure – hadn't been reached yet.

That's been the hardest so far: watching our seven-year-old daughter decline steadily over the last five months. While the rate of decline was now decreasing, the last operation certainly didn't help. What's more, we were not sure what proton beam would bring in the short term and long term: fatigue, certainly, but also possible cognitive decline over years (a slow death?), further damage of hormonal functions and therefore possibly physical aptitudes. Who knew? Not us. Not now, in any case, though the realisation that proton beam was not your regular aspirin-taking cure was not long in coming.

What we did know was that there is no secret formula in life – no magic wand. Grace does not rain equally from the high good. It was going to take sustained effort and focus, over probably eighteen to twenty-four months, to gradually rebuild Millie through small, cumulative improvements. We still had to start growth hormone replacement therapy. That was going to have an effect on her, hopefully for the better, but you can never tell. And both Vanessa and I are fully committed to see this through, whatever it takes. I was convinced that if Millie was going to survive cancer, there was much hope for a full, long and satisfying life. Sure, there would be some boundaries, but then who doesn't have boundaries in life? It was going to take time and effort, but we'd get there.

We still hadn't got to the bottom of the night-time feeding, which was still happening despite our best efforts to keep some foods out of reach. Millie would just switch preference from fruit bars, breadsticks, popcorn, crisps. We even discussed the possibility of putting a lock on the kitchen door. But we were also aware that Millie might still be going through a period of adjustment and we did not want to rush into making changes too quickly. We felt that we would deal with this issue in time, but much like GOSH, we wanted to see proton beam therapy through first.

We are leaving for Oklahoma City this morning. How do you pack for two months away from home? More easily than two weeks away, we discovered. Two months away shifts your mind-set from trying to take home with you to accepting that you'll have to rely on your new environment to make do. You can't pack for every eventuality, food-wise and clothes-wise, when you go away for two months, and the fact there is no choice means there is a new-found freedom. That was liberating in many ways and made the process of packing three suitcases much more enjoyable than it normally is (i.e. Vanessa putting things in and me taking them out).

I also upgraded our tickets to business class. We don't normally travel business class, as I've never understood the point of it, whether or not you can afford it. Surely anything is tolerable up to a certain number of hours, especially when you're a grown up. I could never justify paying five to ten times more for the pleasure of a bit more legroom or more frequent meals. Add to this the fact that we are five whenever we travel, so even EasyJet ends up costing thousands – you get the picture. This was different, however. Millie needed to be comfortable so I felt it was much more justifiable. Actually, it turned out to be completely worth it.

Our taxi arrives. We all get in. As we drive away, the children say goodbye to our house. We say goodbye to Didda, our housekeeper, nanny and friend all in one, who is here today to see us off. She's been a great support over the last five months – thank you, Didda!

We're leaving for our Oklahoman adventure. First stop Heathrow. Millie utters the last cheerio to the front gate, and so said, turns toward the Heaven her face.

# SO DREW FULL MORE THAN
# THOUSAND SPLENDOURS
# TOWARD US

*4) Day 157 – Sunday 8th September*

I get a call from Anna on my way to Heathrow to wish me luck and courage in this last intensive phase of treatment. I have known Anna for eight years, and have worked closely with her for much of that period. We are now business partners in our small start-up. Anna has been extremely supportive over the last five months, and she will continue to be while I focus on Millie's radiotherapy treatment. She has provided invaluable backing and encouragement, and I feel fortunate to work with one of the most principled, loyal people I know. I don't tell her all that on the phone – but now I wish I had.

What she knew but didn't tell me, so as not to ruin my already stressful seventeen-hour trip to the States, was that our third business partner had just resigned. I would get an email from him the following morning. I personally would not have chosen that specific channel of communication; though I understand the decision to leave, and telling me about it was probably made harder by my own personal situation. I'm not upset about his decision to go – his life is his own to make choices about. He has my full support and I wish him luck in his new venture.

We get to Heathrow without a problem. Our first flight takes us to Washington, as there are no direct flights to Oklahoma City. From Washington we would take a connecting flight to Oklahoma Will Rogers World Airport. The flight to Washington goes without a hitch. All my children (and secretly, me) love business class and it makes a huge difference. Even Luca Jack, who is four, manages to stay put for the full eight hours watching his iPad, or the TV monitor provided, or playing on his reclining seat. My eldest loves it even more (bad omen) and begs me to book the same on the way back. Advice to parents of a child with cancer travelling to the US for treatment: if business class is a remotely affordable luxury, it is worth spending the money on that, and going for a cheaper hotel, as most hotels in Oklahoma are when compared to London. I guess everything probably is, when compared to London.

I get slightly worried when one of the American flight attendants asks me where we're heading. "Oklahoma City? Nobody goes to Oklahoma City! What on earth are you going there for?" It's always difficult to give an answer without making people feel unnecessarily embarrassed.

I look out of the plane window. All is still and calm. It's such a contrast to the turbulence blasting inside my head, where so many doubts about Millie and the outcome of her cure remain.


*5) Day 157 – Sunday 8th September*

Still Sunday. With the time difference, it is proving difficult to move from today; a day that's getting longer and longer. Going to Oklahoma feels just as prolonged.

I manage to watch a movie (a rare occurrence these days). It's *The Internship,* with Vince Vaughn and Owen Wilson playing two salesmen whose careers have been torpedoed by the digital age. They find their way on to a coveted internship at Google, where they must compete with a group of young, tech-savvy geniuses for a shot at employment. It's brilliant and exactly the kind of distraction I need.

We land in Washington, and the most painful part of our journey starts: US immigration and waiting for a connecting flight. This is made worse as it's getting late (UK time is approximately 7pm), we are travelling with three young children and because one of them has just gone to hell and back. I should have given this more thought. I know the airline offered a wheelchair (Millie wasn't keen) but what I failed to do was see if there was a way to speed up the immigration process by giving advance warning of our arrival (I suspect there isn't). I doubt it would have made much difference. I had travelled to the US before, but immigration is less painful when you travel on your own. The queue is huge – like a mass of senseless beasts, or perhaps that's just how we're being treated.

We have to go through immigration declaring if we have any item of 'food' or 'fruit'. We are travelling with three children over a fifteen-hour period, so of course we've got fucking food and fruit. And arguably one is a subsection of another, so I'm not sure why both are listed. In a rash of ill-advised honesty, I had ticked the 'food and fruit' box on the little immigration slip. I shouldn't have. When 99% of people go straight through, we are asked to step aside and, treated like drug dealers, are stripped of the offending and felonious items of food. There were three ham sandwiches, one for each of the three children – one with cancer – that we had prepared for the wait of our connecting flight, and three apples as a healthy snack for the flight itself. I am helpfully told by a US immigration official, as she throws my food items away (a US official that did not make eye contact once, or smile for that matter), that "We've got food in this country too". I'll be sure to look for it, and for a sense of humour too. Or is that humanity? Charity? Compassion? Empathy? I would find plenty of that, just not in the immigration lounge of Washington DC. There was none there, when there really should have been.

*6) Day 157 – Sunday 8th September*

Millie is struggling. We eventually get to the boarding gate for our connecting flight to Oklahoma City but there's still a couple of hours to go. By now we're all tired and blurriness has set in.

We finally board. The flight is only a couple of hours long and we will be met at the airport by the patient services manager. It's been a long day. As we approach Oklahoma City in the night sky, I notice high, slim, upright stakes with red lights at regular intervals from the top, all the way down (I later learn they are communication masts). There seems to be hundreds, as if partly suspended above the ground. As we approach Will Rogers Airport, these thousands of splendours draw increasingly nearer towards us. Touch down. We have arrived at our final destination.

# LET THE DESTINED YEARS
# COME ROUND

*7) Day 159 – Tuesday 10th September am*

We spent most of yesterday, our first day here, visiting two housing options, both in the north of Oklahoma City, in a neighbourhood called Edmonds. Paula, Linda's sister and in real estate, as luck would have it, has been kind enough to take us to both properties. One was sourced by her prior to our arrival and one was sourced by ProCure. As one of the properties isn't furnished, Paula has also contacted furniture rental companies, and has come with me to help fill out paperwork at the estate agents. This is someone I met for the first time in Oklahoma – doesn't know me or Millie, and is taking time out of her work day to help us! She has also spent many hours prior to this, planning for the trip and our arrival, all out of the goodness of her heart. I am so grateful to Paula, to Linda and soon to Mary – they validate all that is good in us humans. I am just ashamed I have never done anything similar for anyone in my life, not in the way they are doing for me now. I don't know if I would have in the past, but I know how I will repay the kindness that has been afforded to me and my family: I hope I have the opportunity to help others when I find myself on the other side of the equation.

We should find out later today if the house we put an offer on will be accepted. Meanwhile, we go to the ProCure Proton Therapy Centre for the first time. It is a relatively recent addition to the Oklahoma City landscape, having opened in July 2009, and is only one of a handful of centres in the US to treat tumours with proton therapy, an advanced form of radiation therapy. The centre itself is a vast modern building of some 60,000 sq ft, containing four treatment rooms designed to treat different types of tumours. Each patient (or family, where the patient is a child) is assigned a personal care team, which includes a physician, nurse, radiation therapists and treatment team assistants who stay with the family throughout the treatment. We will meet a few of them tomorrow – today is more about induction and meeting the support team, including the receptionists. We are shown where the coffee machine is, where the pharmacy is, we are given a US mobile phone, two rental cars have been organised for us; one was delivered to our hotel yesterday morning and one will be collected for us later in the week. Customer service at its best! And it's a proton beam centre!

It feels like a mix of a first day at work and the beginning of a holiday of sorts. The atmosphere is jovial, cleanliness is evident, and nothing in the reception area, or the rooms we are shown, give any indication that this is a medical facility. Even the WiFi is free and super-fast, as it is in most places you go to in Oklahoma City – supermarkets, shopping malls, bookshops, museums. Everything smacks of a customer-centric commercial facility, they just sell a different kind of product, or products: protons for those who can afford it, or those who have medical insurance.

It is our first experience of healthcare outside of the UK and, from a user perspective, far more pleasant. Of course,

I'm not comparing like with like, but a visit to the children's hospital later this week would provide a similar feeling, and it's the only hospital I have ever been to that has valet parking for its patients. Not that we haven't been served well by GOSH – the team there saved my daughter's eyesight and hopefully her life. The level of excellence is irrefutable, but GOSH is an NHS facility and suffers from the culture and philosophy of a system based on free healthcare for all supported by chronic underinvestment, as opposed to private investment. Of course, the NHS doesn't let 16% of ill people die every year because they don't have health insurance, so I know which system I would chose. But I do think the UK has much to learn from the way the US has been able to adapt the customer-centric approach of their service industry to a patient-centric approach in these private medical institutions. It's a convergence of culture – mixed, actually, with deep religious undertones (the only peculiar element). ProCure is a strange animal in that sense, part hospital, part cult. Staff are deeply dedicated to the cause and many of them have had personal experience of cancer. They have a clear visceral affiliation with ProCure and an unwavering commitment to its vision and values.

The sign on the entrance door says that smoking and carrying firearms is prohibited on campus. You know you're in the States when a facility dedicated to curing cancer feels the need to remind its patients that carrying a gun is not permitted in the building. The patient service manager confirms that tomorrow we will have our first appointment with the radiologist, who will make a treatment plan for Millie. This is the person who will ensure the beams are positioned such that future risks of recurrence are minimised and, hopefully, guide Millie towards a complete resurrection.

I get an email from Linda via the super-fast ProCure WiFi connection. After some thought, Mary would like to offer us the possibility of renting her house for a couple of months. It's in Nichols Hills (our preference), so would we be free to go and meet her later today at, say, 5pm, to have a look at her home? Of course we would.

*8) Day 159 – Tuesday 10th September: pm*

After a couple of hours of meeting and greeting at the centre, we head back into town, or Whole Foods to be precise. We use this organic supermarket extensively during this initial phase as the only place we have lunch and dinner (until we get permanent accommodation). We had been going to the one in London since it opened, so finding a Whole Foods in Oklahoma gives us an extra sense of security somehow. I never thought a supermarket could do that. We only have time for a quick lunch as we have to go and meet with Casady's director of admission.

Casady is a great campus-style school. We are greeted by the headmaster and the head of the lower division, and we spend a good two hours visiting each department. The reception couldn't have been warmer, more sincere or heartfelt. I felt an immediate connection with Casady that would only strengthen as the weeks went by. We agree on a start date (16th September, so next Monday) and we buy a few items of uniform from their onsite shop. The following day I go and sign various contractual forms and arrange for fees to be paid over. Not that paying diminishes the gesture extended by Casady in any way. I was always fully expecting to pay fees.

It's getting to be a busy day. Millie is struggling but we still have one more stop – an important one – and that is meeting Mary, the lady who is going to show us her home, and be generous enough to rent it to us for two months should we want it. Again, this would entail a tenancy agreement and payment of market rent, but again, it does not devalue the immense gesture this lady is prepared to extend to us. To go away for two months and rent us her home, which she has never rented to anybody else before, all because she had heard of Millie through Linda. She herself had cared for a cancer patient (the amazing power of empathy) and was compassionate enough to know that it would make a material difference to us as a family. How do you repay something like that? We find out later that Linda and (possibly) Mary also may have had some influence over encouraging Casady to be flexible enough to consider our case. We think they knew someone closely involved with the school.

The house is lovely, in *the* neighbourhood we want to be in (close to Whole Foods and Casady, amongst other things) and only twelve minutes' drive to ProCure. The centre would have adopted a different strategy. They prefer people to be close by, the theory being that you have to get to the centre every day for treatment. But treatments only last thirty minutes, and once they are done, we feel it is better to be more central and closer to useful amenities, especially as we'll have a daily school run for our two other children. Eventually, Millie will actually be well enough to start school in the mornings and Casady would be thoughtful enough to offer that as a gesture of goodwill.

Anyway, we couldn't ask for a better solution than to rent Mary's house while we are in Oklahoma City. The lane it is on even happens to feature in one of my favourite plays. It has the same name as the lane where an infamous flower girl used to live before starting elocution lessons with one Professor Higgins. I could have danced all night... We all agree to proceed with the transaction, so to speak, and aim for next Tuesday as the move-in date. Wow! Thanks Dom, my old mate, for introducing me to Linda. The investment made during those countless drunken nights when we were in our twenties has finally paid off! Thanks Linda for introducing me to Mary and Paula, and thank you ladies for the amazing difference you have made to the life of little Millie May. I will be forever grateful for your kindness, compassion and remarkable human qualities.

Today was a good day. Much was achieved, and this would put us in good stead for the remainder of our stay. A Kung Fu teacher called Sifu J (*teacher J*), who later in our stay was kind enough to offer my children Kung Fu lessons (his wife having also been diagnosed with a brain tumour) always taught his class to work hard at practising first time round, because it makes things easier later on. Hard now means easy later. And so it was with the investment in planning and nurturing of relationships that had been made in the month prior to coming to Oklahoma City.

Today we visited the centre for the first time, secured a great house for the next two months and received confirmation that our two healthy children could start school next week. And all gift-wrapped with love from fellow human beings – who were strangers until a few weeks ago – as if directly instructed by Venus herself.

*9) Day 160 – Wednesday 11th September*

We have been dreading today since Dr C confirmed we had been accepted for proton beam in the States, but warned us of 'expectation setting US-style' with regards to short and long-term side effects. She even told us of patients who nearly took the next plane back home because of it. We are due to meet the ProCure nurse and radiologist and they will talk us through proton beam and what it entails (i.e. they will set expectations). This is when the nice doctors take you aside to sign consent forms and go through the list of lovely things that will/may/could happen in the short or long term as a result of the treatment. The worst we have had so far was the second such conversation with Millie's neurosurgeon just before her first operation. So we feel relatively prepared for anything that might come our way, but as with all unknowns, we are apprehensive about what we will be told and about those proton beam's side effects that we haven't already read before. We are hoping that there will be more accuracy in the prediction of these – but we'd end up disappointed on that front. We will be spending much of the day at ProCure, as Millie needs to have the MRI (her seventh in just under six months) and CT scans that will be used to plan her treatment.

We meet with D (the nurse) and Dr C, who confusingly has the same surname as the other Dr C at GOSH, though this Dr C is a cordial American chap of Asian descent, wearing a Spider-Man T-shirt. He looks far too young to be one of the two radiology paediatric oncologists at the centre, but that's probably a reflection of my age, as opposed to his. And I'm only forty-one. How will I feel when I'm sixty and meet the equivalent of Dr C? He is also the Dr C that, on review of the MRI scan showing an unidentified blood clot a couple of weeks ago, insisted Millie underwent a third craniotomy in as many months. So he's not my favourite person in the world, it has to be said.

Dr C starts by examining Millie, who is her normal calm

self and no doubt now used to everyone examining her in the same way over the last six months or so. One of the tests he performs is to check her peripheral vision. He puts each of his hands level to the left and right of Millie's eyes, and asks Millie to identify which fingers he is wiggling: left, right, neither or both, whilst she is looking at his nose. She does brilliantly – not a single mistake and assured in her answer (for Millie, that means being very confident of it being the right answer). Dr C confirms that while vision does sometimes return in cases similar to Millie's, it is very rare indeed for the visual field to have regained so much width since the operation and loss of sight.

We don't have a formal assessment by ophthalmology at GOSH until December, but seeing Millie doing so well in tests relating to eyesight never ceases to cheer me up. I could watch her pass eye examinations all day long. Ultimately, what pleases me the most (an understatement…) is that her eyes and optic nerves have regained the ability to see. It will make such a gigantic difference to her quality of life if she survives cancer. Dr C finishes his examination and proceeds to tell us a little more about the side effects of proton beam therapy generally, and those related to irradiating the specific area (tumour bed) where Millie's tumour was located. Yippee!

The goal of all radiation therapy is to destroy tumour cells and prevent regrowth, while protecting the healthy tissue that surrounds the tumour. This is especially important for young children like Millie, as their developing brains and bodies are extremely sensitive to the potential long-term effects of radiation. Millie no longer has a tumour, but in order to minimise the risks of recurrence, Dr C, by comparing various MRI scans and undertaking a variety of calculations, will irradiate the tumour bed as well as a one-centimetre circumference around it. One centimetre is quite a lot, it is effectively a cube of 2x2cm healthy cells (there's no tumour left in there) that will be irradiated beyond repair to ensure that whatever rogue malignant cells left, post surgery and chemotherapy, cease indefinitely to be. As those healthy cells are located in Millie's head, they are, quite literally, brain matter. And in her case, take up most of her pituitary and some of her hypothalamus. Luckily, we are told later that the hypothalamus is not particularly sensitive to radiotherapy. I had already been told that by Millie's oncologist at GOSH, Dr H, but it is always reassuring when unconnected medical professionals corroborate snippets of information in this way. It makes it more plausible, and more likely to be true. So the pituitary gland will 'get it', as will the regions of the brain that are in the path of the proton beam.

More on the physics of protons later, but broadly, proton beam can be managed such that the entry dose is 25% of the dose normally required with regular photons to irradiate the tumour bed. This is because protons release most of their energy in a very specific way, in a very specific site, which, luckily for Millie, can be calculated with precision. Unlike photons, they do not have an exit dose, so they effectively 'die' once all energy has been released. Therefore whilst the side effects associated with entry doses are much lesser than those associated with conventional (photon) radiotherapy, they can occur with proton too. They are just far less likely and not as marked, perceptible or conspicuous as they would be with photons.

OK, so here we go in terms of side effects – the good, the bad and the ugly. Actually, in the context of the treatment Millie has had so far, only the bad and the ugly ever turn up:

- **General short-term side effects (i.e. temporary)**: These we are not worried about – they include tiredness, skin irritation, hair loss in the treated area, nausea and headaches. As far as Millie is concerned, the site of the tumour is such that Dr C does not expect any temporary hair loss, and any skin irritation ought to be very mild. These would have been the two most bothersome side effects for Millie and she won't have them, so that's good. Most of the headaches and nausea is expected in the first week of treatment if at all, and fatigue is normally encountered in the last two weeks of treatment and lasts for approximately a month afterwards, but is nothing an afternoon nap isn't able to redress. Slightly more concerning is when Dr C tells us that sometimes, the short-term side effect of proton beam therapy is to aggravate the initial symptoms that arose when the tumour was first diagnosed. This is because it irritates the part that has already been damaged. In Millie's case, that's eyesight, but given how well she has recovered from that perspective, he doesn't anticipate this to be of any functional concern (and again, it may well not happen).

- **Long-term side effects (i.e. permanent)**: These are the ones that are most concerning for us. Radiation can decrease the ability of the pituitary gland to produce certain hormones. The hypothalamus, as we are told, is very sensitive to surgery but significantly less so to radiation. The risk of hormone deficiencies is very low immediately following radiation, but gradually increases over the years. Some patients develop hormone deficiencies a year or two after radiation, while others may have normal levels for ten or twenty years and then develop low hormone levels.

In a way, this is almost irrelevant for Millie because the tumour damaged the area normally affected by radiotherapy. She already has diabetes insipidus, and it is *very* likely she will require growth hormones – we are due to kick-start that particular process in November when we are back from Oklahoma. The uncertain one is ACTH, the hormone responsible for stimulating the adrenals to produce cortisol (I spoke at length about this one in Part II). It is the one causing us the most angst, as Millie is taking hydrocortisone now as a precautionary measure, until we can establish one way or another if she is able to produce her own. Radiotherapy may well mean she ends up requiring hydrocortisone for the rest of her life. Given the notoriously damaging side effects of this particular drug, this prospect doesn't fill us with joy, and it is also the drug we are currently blaming (probably wrongly) for Millie's rapid weight gain.

In addition to the endocrine function, the entry dose, while significantly lower than conventional radiotherapy, still means that one of the possible side effects is the gradual loss of cognition over time. Quantifiably, this represents a small loss of IQ over years. The truth is that no precise measure actually exists, because comparative proton beam studies involving children (as a study group) are not readily available. Proton beam for this type of tumour is a relatively new thing, and children that may have received proton beam back in the mid-1990s would be in their late twenties now for example. The side effects also vary depending on the location of the tumour. There is one study that actually suggests proton beam therapy may spare cognitive functioning – or in any case enable IQ to remain generally stable for the first three years post-radiation therapy, and then decrease only very slightly. We don't know what happens next as it hasn't yet been measured in that particular, and very recent, study. In contrast, photon is associated with significant cognitive risk, with IQ scores declining by more than half a standard deviation (I think that's about two points per annum) with each additional year post photon therapy. So Millie might have difficulty with abstract subjects like maths and physics over time. Well, neither her father nor her mother was particularly gifted in those subjects either and they are able to engage with the outside world relatively well (or as awkwardly as most), so we can live with that uncertainty. The final side effect is the risk of developing a second malignancy due to the proton beam affecting healthy cells, though this is far less risky than it would have been with traditional photon radiation. There is little to be done on this one. It comes with the territory of curing cancer.

So overall, our chat turned out to be not so bad. The only two risks, as far as Millie is concerned, are cognitive decline and a second malignancy. The latter is so unquantifiable it's not worth thinking about at this stage (besides, there is nothing we can do at this stage to mitigate this risk). The cognitive decline may or may not occur, and if it does, it will be so minimal as to be functionally non-perceptive (we hope...). And we won't know for another ten to twenty years, because proton beam therapy for this specific type of tumour only started relatively recently.

I say let the destined years come round! We're doing well if we ever get to find out.

# O FOND ANXIETY OF
# MORTAL MEN

*10) Day 161 – Thursday 12th September*

Part of the process of integration includes registering at the local children's hospital (the one with valet parking). Our nurse from ProCure comes to the hotel to pick us up and show us the way for this first time (what a lovely touch!), although TomTom seems to know where it's going. We are registering with the local oncology consultant. Not because Millie needs further chemotherapy, thank God, but just in case and also for regular sodium and blood test checks that continue to be necessary. We regurgitate for the umpteenth time the events of the last five months, and the oncologist, like everyone else before her, does a few tests, including peripheral vision. She confirms that Millie has been very lucky indeed to regain so much of her eyesight, and so much width in her field of vision.

We also talk about protocol and radiation therapy. She somewhat confuses us initially by suggesting Millie is part of a trial (huh… no one mentioned anything to us) but then we discover that in the US, children with Millie's condition have the brain and the whole spine irradiated – whereas UK protocol only focuses on the area of the tumour and tumour bed. That's reassuring, and I'm delighted we are under the care of GOSH. Actually, I'm delighted to be able to pick from the best of both worlds. This particular confusion also prompts her to share with us a scholarly article relating to the main findings of the trial that gave rise to PEI protocol in the first place, the chemotherapy protocol Millie has undertaken.

This is the first time someone from the medical profession has shared trial results in printed form, so I'm a little anxious about what I am going to read. The abstract dates back to 1997 and starts: 'Secreting germ cells tumours are an invariably *fatal* subgroup within the malignant paediatric brain tumours'. In other words, had Millie been diagnosed prior to this trial, her chances of survival would have been minimal. It then goes on to explain that as a result of this, an international work group was set up to cooperate in a study for diagnosis and treatment of such tumours, and ran a pilot protocol which then became PEI. The results (I feel a rush of adrenaline) are thus (this is where having a summary becomes less helpful): Patients in the study were aged eight to nineteen. Seven children were diagnosed by elevated tumour markers. In six patients, the tumour is primarily resected (i.e. removed by surgery) and two children are biopsied. In two children, spinal metastases are diagnosed initially. Tumour marker response (*this is where it gets interesting*) is evaluated in sixteen children. Thirteen out of sixteen patients show a clear marker normalisation after two courses of PEI (*the chemo Millie has had, and the response Millie has had – I am now slightly annoyed at GOSH's oncologist for not being more frank in his prediction at the beginning of treatment. He did say this cancer is sensitive to chemotherapy, but he certainly didn't say that the chances of this happening were very favourable at 82%)*. Following completion of chemotherapy, further operations where required, and radiotherapy, seventeen out of nineteen patients were still alive at the time of writing; sixteen of them in complete remission with a median follow up of eleven months. One of the original nineteen died after a spinal relapse following his fourth course of PEI (*Millie's cancer hadn't spread to her spine, thankfully*). And one died post-operatively because of tumour bleeding (*again, didn't happen to Millie*). So, actually, the relevant sample for Millie has to be seventeen – and out of those seventeen, sixteen are in complete remission. That's 94% survival at the eleven-month point.

We need to be cautious not to run away with optimism: eleven months ain't five years, and what Millie has is a very serious illness. Still, I think this study shows that Millie is in a very good place indeed, given where she was six months ago. Despite myself, I feel we can probably nudge the 65% we were told about at the beginning of our treatment a little further towards 70% or perhaps 75%. I didn't think much about percentages at the beginning of Millie's illness because nothing had yet crystallised. We didn't know if her cancer was going to be sensitive to chemotherapy (it was) and we didn't know if surgery was able to remove little, much or all of the tumour (it removed all of it). But now we *know*. It has happened, and I can't help but feel we can let ourselves think slightly more optimistically than a mere 'two out of three' chance.

Oh fond anxiety of mortal men... I do not believe mine will subside until I've lived through the next three years at least, no matter what probability you throw at me.

Nearly a week has gone past since we arrived in Oklahoma City (also known as OKC) and it has gone very quickly. We seem to have adjusted to living in a hotel relatively well. We adjusted to the time difference the very first night (it was a long trip though…) and we have established an enjoyable routine of breakfast at the hotel and then lunch and dinner at Whole Foods (it has a good variety of cooked meals, salads and sushi, and a pleasant room with tables to go and eat it). Besides, it is *very* hot in OKC and the weather is certainly helping us to adopt a relaxed lifestyle (we haven't seen a cloud for six days). People in OKC are laid-back and welcoming. Even driving is pleasant. It's all very moderate, no horn, no traffic, no tailgating, constant speed limits everywhere (20mph in the whole of the neighbourhood we will end up living).

It's not a holiday, don't get me wrong, we're here for one reason and one reason only – to cure Millie of cancer – but actually, this experience will turn out to be significantly more positive than a holiday. A lot of it has to do with the length of time we're here for. We decide to explore like tourists, and, starting with the OKC Zoo today, and the Science Museum tomorrow, over the next two months, we visit many local attractions and museums, which all of us end up enjoying. OKC actually has greater depths of culture than I expected and, as it turns out, than some of the locals thought, too.

OKC Zoo was recently voted as one of the best US zoos and it deserves the title. To start with, it's huge and clean, and devoid of crowds, unlike London Zoo, for example. It's also only five minutes away from the centre of town, as most things in OKC would turn out to be. It's a perfect opportunity for Millie to do some exercise. She is still slowly putting on weight, and managing her intake of food is a constant effort. It helps being in a hotel with no fridge or larder. She manages a good ten minutes of walking, and for the first time in ages even tries to climb into a tree house and cross a wobbly bridge in the zoo's playground. We have a buggy with us though, and it proves useful for some of the excursion. Now and again, Millie can leave the safety of her seated position to explore her surroundings, and then go back and have a rest, and so on.

The same happens at the Science Museum (more science attraction park than museum, but enjoyable nonetheless). Millie even manages to go on a Segway – the scooter with two wheels, and the one you can't fall off. She actually does rather well. She loves it, of course. She hasn't managed to engage in activities with Ellie and Luca for a long time – well, since 5th April really – and being in OKC actually forces us to include her. Her attendance is compulsory, as we can't leave her at the hotel on her own. But she does brilliantly.

If I think back to 7th April, when she woke up blind from her first brain operation with an uncertain prognosis, and the fact she has since gone through a further two brain operations and four cycles of chemotherapy, it is, quite simply, miraculous that she is able to follow us at all, albeit a little slower than my other two. She keeps up with the pace we are setting. Yes, she uses the buggy now and then; yes, she stays in it when the other two swing off monkey bars, as if gravity was somehow reversed, but she's here with us, walking, talking, eating (a bit too much), seeing and being. I remind myself of that every time I feel down about seeing her still so weak.

Recovery will be a long process but we're doing well, and keeping Millie close to the flock, to us as a family, is helping her challenge herself a little more than if we had just come here with her.

## 12) Day 166 – Tuesday 17th September

Ellie and Luca started school yesterday. They were a little apprehensive going in and didn't enjoy their first day, but by the end of the week, both adjusted better than we could ever have expected. Casady made such an effort to integrate them both during the first week. We feel privileged to be treated in such a way, and grateful to the school for going the extra mile in order to make our stay more comfortable, and for trying so hard to ensure my two healthy children feel welcome and appreciated.

Being in a different school would turn out to be such a positive learning experience. It wasn't on the curriculum for maths and English back at home, but significantly more valuable nonetheless. There is much to be said about this, and experiencing a different schooling environment makes more noticeable the unrelenting exam-driven arms race that seems to have possessed the UK schooling system over the last two decades. The focus is on exam results and an appetite for wonder is no longer part of the curriculum. Reading a book because you enjoy reading it, rather than because it's on the syllabus, seems to have become an alien concept. Learning for the pleasure of learning is fast becoming extinct and it's a tragedy. Perhaps we'll have to look elsewhere for our children's education, but for now, we must concentrate on the task at hand.

When we pick the children up from school today, we actually drive back to Mary's house. It's 'moving in' day, and tonight we sleep in what will be our home for the next two months.

We get a call from ProCure confirming that Millie's plan has been finalised and that she will start her first session of therapy on 23rd September.

Millie inducted into ProCure: tick! Ellie and Luca in a US school while Millie has her treatment: tick! New plug-and-play home, in the best neighbourhood we could ask for, rented for the rest of our stay: tick!

Day eight of OKC and we're set. I'm very proud of us, even if this sentiment is a somewhat self-indulgent and narcissistic double rainbow.

# WITH LIVELY RAY
# SERENE OVERCOME
# THE MASSIEST AIR

*13) Day 169 – Friday 20th September*

Part of the induction at ProCure is to attend a tour of the
facilities and a lunch with other new patients (or should that
be customers?). A tour and a lunch! We meet one of the
patient services managers, who guides us though several rooms
of the centre, much like a tour guide. We see the consulting
rooms where Millie will be assessed once a week by her
allocated (dedicated!) nurse and radiation oncologist; we go
through the room where children who cannot lie still are
woken up after general anaesthetic (luckily this won't happen
to Millie); and we are brought to the meeting rooms and
conference rooms with various white boards filled with
equations. There is much physics involved in proton beam
therapy, and this is where plans are finalised to ensure protons
release energy in the right way. It's also where we meet people
with job titles like 'dosimetrist' – the person responsible for
ensuring the calibrations and functionality of medical
equipment used in radiation therapy is working properly; also
'medical physicist' – all professions I never knew existed.

Perhaps the most impressive room of the tour is the treatment room itself, where the so-called gantry resides. Think MRI scan on a grand scale. The gantry is a huge cylindrical room, with a crane-like nozzle coming out of it, and a semi-suspended bed in the bore of the gantry itself. The nozzle is fitted with customised dose-shaping devices – circular brass plates the size of dinner plates, about two inches thick, with a hole in the centre shaped in the outline of a target (usually the tumour or the tumour bed). These plates are used to block the proton beam outside a specified safety margin, and are also used to adjust the penetration depth of the protons that pass through the aperture. This enables the team to shape the beam to match a very specific 3D area of Millie's tumour bed and also to adjust how deep they want the proton to penetrate before it releases its energy (Braggs' peak – more on that later). Every single patient has their own customised brass plate fitted by a team of people called 'machinists'. And there is a very specific, secure protocol to ensure the right plate is used for the right patient.

The bed itself (where Millie lay earlier today for her trial run) moves so as to position the patient in a very specific way, and much of the daily thirty-minute irradiation session is spent doing just that: positioning and immobilising. Yes, there's a job title for that too – it's the 'immobilisation specialist'. In addition to lying still on a bed, Millie will also wear a made-to-measure mask. This is a silicon-looking mask with hundreds of little holes in it, like a rigid head-shaped plastic net. The delivery of the proton beam itself lasts only a few minutes. I don't really understand the technology, or the physics behind it, but it is mind blowing. And there are currently centres in construction that take this to an even greater level of precision. I think it is called pencil beam and I have no doubt that within the next few decades, humankind will be able to deliver, on a grand scale and cheaply, single protons targeted towards single cancerous cells; or perhaps do away with Proton Beam altogether by applying targeted viral attacks on cancerous cells. Who knows…

One of the rooms we don't get to see is the cyclotron accelerator, and it must be "truly awesome", as my Oklahoman carer would say. This machine lives deep in the bowels of the centre and is responsible for generating the proton beam in the first instance, which is then directed, through various positioning of magnets, towards each of the four treatment rooms they have at ProCure. From each, these lively rays of serene enter the patient's body (or in Millie's case, the head) and destroy the most resilient of tumour cells.

The tour finishes in the boardroom, a spacious room with a wall-to-wall glass window overlooking the waiting area below. The story goes that the founders wanted the window there, so those making important decisions in the room were reminded of the primary objective behind ProCure – the wellbeing of those sitting below waiting to be treated. Nice story, if somewhat on the romantic side.

We have lunch and are encouraged to share our stories. There are four other couples there, and most (if not all) are here to cure prostate cancer. Millie is with us during the lunch and we recount our journey matter of factly, as we have done so many times before. We recall the last five months, the blindness, the brain tumour, cancer, the three brain operations, the four cycles of chemotherapy, the kidney failures. And then it happens: one by one, they all come to shake our hand when lunch finishes. They tell us what an extraordinary little girl she is, and how silly they all feel, telling their story about a trivial little prostate cancer. They feel what I felt several times when I encountered (as I often did at GOSH) parents in a much worse situation than I was: humility. It happened to me the last time when I got to know the father of a four-year-old girl suffering from Stage 4 neuroblastoma in Lion Ward. Her treatment, which is to span a year and a half (much of which spent in hospital) makes Millie's condition seem like a bad headache. There are always people worse off, and most of the people I met today have it better, but the focus has been so intense over the last five months that we have lost the ability to step back and feel sorry for ourselves.

We can only look forward, we can only work to sustain the ongoing effort required to make Millie better a little bit at a time, a little bit every day. People coming up to us, reminding us of what we already know (that we've had a rotten time of it in the last five months) doesn't bother me. It gratifies me and reaffirms my commitment to ensure we stay focused for as long as it takes.


*14) Day 172 – Monday 23rd September*


Today has finally arrived. The beginning of the end of cancer treatment for Millie: her very first proton beam session. By now she has had several trial runs, one in the UK and one a few days ago, one dummy mask and one actual mask made up. This is the made-to-measure silicone-type mask used to immobilise Millie during treatment. She knows what's coming, but is still a little apprehensive, as no one else is allowed in through the door with her. Parents and carers need to wait in the reception area while it all happens. I think the apprehension is less to do with going on her own and more to do with the unknown. She hasn't experienced this type of treatment before and I guess she's a little scared – hell, she's seven, I would be too and I'm forty-one. We tell her the worst thing is that it would be a bit boring, you know, having to lie on a bed for half an hour, but I guess there's no substitute for experience... Within a couple of sessions, Millie would understand nothing bad would happen and start enjoying the attention of the amazing nurses who took care of her.

After each session, Millie receives one bead to add to her collection of 'Beads of Courage'. This is worth an explanation. Last week, Millie was given a bag and a bunch of beads marketed as Beads of Courage, along with a daily bead journal. The beads represent each of the treatments, side effects and suffering children with cancer have to go through (chemotherapy, hair loss, radiation, stem cell biopsy, transfusion, lumbar punctures, tests, scans, clinic visits, bone marrow aspirate, injections, line placement, hospital stays, to name but a few). Each bead represents one of those things – red bead for transfusion, black for injection, tortoise for lumbar puncture, purple for infusion and so on and so forth. The beads are a tangible representation of Millie's treatment journey. They are there to record and to tell, but perhaps more importantly for Millie, so that she can *own* her story of courage. The one telling the world that it may have been hard, but she did it. She loves them – and so do I.

As we leave the centre, bright rays of light come shining though the large glass frontage along which the reception area is laid out. My eyes follow them up towards the horizon. It's another sunny day in Oklahoma City.


*15) Day 176 – Friday 27th September*


There have been a lot of firsts for Millie over the last few weeks, as she has begun to regain strength, energy and stamina.

This morning is the first time she's been to school since March (Easter break – when it all began). Casady has kindly agreed to take her for mornings only. In order to make it easy on Millie, the school has suggested kindergarten to ensure she can reintegrate into a classroom environment without worrying too much about the curriculum (who cares about maths and English). She is not as apprehensive as I thought she would be, and definitely not as much as the other two on their first day, that's for sure. She's mostly keen. Keen to go in and experience what she hasn't had the chance to experience in five long months of gruelling cancer treatment. Keen to engage with peers, with other little girls. Keen to embrace new learning experiences. And, mostly I think, keen to feel normal again.

There are no words to describe how I feel today, and the level of gratitude I feel towards Casady and its teachers for being flexible enough to make this happen. It means everything to Millie to be able to go to the same school as Luca and Ellie, and wear the same uniform. Therefore it means everything to me and Vanessa. We would start by picking her up at 11:30am, but by the end of it she was doing the full half-day, staying until just after lunch. I am sure it would also help Millie through treatment – most of the children undergoing proton beam therapy do little other than spend thirty minutes at the centre during their allocated slots. Six weeks and thirty sessions is a long time for a seven-year-old when there is little else to do.

Being in a classroom environment at Casady doing fun stuff, can only promote progress and healing – at every level: physical (she's trying new things in the playground, more and more often), mental (she's rediscovering her love of maths, but in a fun, Montessori kind of way) and, most importantly, emotional (she is remembering what it feels like to play with girls her own age and make new friends).

From the martyrdom of cancer, from blindness, from anguish and despair, Millie and our family have found new peace. Who knew we would find it here, in Oklahoma City, of all places?

# LIKE A GOLDEN MIRROR
# IN THE SUN

*16) Day 180 – Tuesday 1st October*

Millie has now undergone six sessions of proton beam. We were told to expect possible headaches and nausea the first week. Millie has had a couple of headaches, but a regular dose of paracetamol was all that was required to get rid of them. She has taken to her new routine very well. She goes to school every morning, has lunch with me and Vanessa, normally at Whole Foods, and then she has her treatment in the afternoon. ProCure runs a specific schedule with regards to the gantry she is on, so as to fit people in accordance to the size of the brass plates, and in such a way that the machinists only need to adjust the gantry fractionally, and in one direction only.

Every time we walk into ProCure, we feel a sense of gratitude towards the consultants at GOSH that have made it possible for us to be here; for Millie to receive the most advanced cancer treatment available, and to be in the best possible shape for it (i.e. in complete remission). It is a shame the UK does not offer it yet, though a couple of centres are due to open towards the end of the decade. It's odd it has taken so long to build one, given the other centres of medical excellence in the UK, and also considering that proton beam has actually been around since 1954, when the first patients were treated. Over the last fifty years only a handful of facilities have become available worldwide, five or six of which are located in the US. One of proton beam's greatest challenges has been, and continues to be, that of cost and accessibility. Building and running a proton beam facility is significantly more expensive than doing the same for conventional photon radiation. So what's the difference? Well, it all lies in the physics of it, and it's been a fascinating area to explore.

Traditionally, external beam radiation has been the standard of care for radiation therapy. Photon beam X-rays (parcels of waves are called photons – like light waves and much the same thing except a different place on the spectrum) are created using two-dimensional models to design the radiation field. Unlike protons, photons enter the patient at a specific site and the dose administered initially increases over the first few centimetres; it then decreases exponentially until it exits the patient. In other words, the entire path of the photon, from the point of entry, through the target site and out the exit site, is irradiated.

Protons, on the other hand, are very different. They are positively charged elementary particles found in the nucleus of every atom in the universe. For proton beam, hydrogen atoms are used (presumably because it's the simplest atom and there's lots of it around, but I might be wrong), with one electron removed. Proton beams enter the patient from several sites, conforming to the exact shape of the target, with the use of the brass plate to shape the beam in several ways. Protons typically release energy (unlike photons) in increasing amounts as they start to slow down, because the slower they move the more atoms they have time to hit, or something to that effect.

When protons stop moving, they release most of their energy in one giant burst of radiation (called a Bragg peak). After that burst, there's very little energy left and they just stop – so there is no 'exit dose' of radiation like there is in X-ray therapy. So the greatest dose of radiation is therefore neither lost at the entry site nor distributed amongst healthy tissue. By altering dose and velocity, the medical team is able to shape the beam so as to minimise the entry dose and ensure that the burst of energy happens at the specific location that is required. For a like-for-like dosage of radiation, the entry dose for proton beam is 25% of what it would be for photons. It's all significantly more complicated than that, of course, because different tissues have different densities and affect protons in a different way.

For Millie, in order to calculate the right dose at the Bragg peak, consideration has been given to protons needing to travel through skin, skull and not just brain, but the various elements that make it up, including right and left hemisphere, hypothalamus, pituitary gland, optic nerve and chiasm etc. That's what the initial plan is there to do: to establish how much, how often and in how many different entry sites.

Millie will have a total target dose of 54.0 CGE (cobalt gray equivalent – the unit of radiation for proton – gray being the unit of radiation for conventional photon radiotherapy). So her thirty sessions will effectively be divided up as follows:

- Fourteen sessions every other day, in two separate beams delivering 1.8 CGE (25.2 CGE in total).
- Fourteen sessions every other alternate day, in two separate beams (in a different location and entry to the ones above) delivering 1.8 CGE (25.2 CGE in total).

- And then two booster sessions at 1.8 CGE each. These are two different 'conedown' fields to spare the dose to the optic structures that tolerate protons less well.

The total of which equals 54.0 CGE, delivered through five or six different access points in order to minimise possible side effects of the entry dose, whilst still delivering 100% of the dosage to the site itself. If you imagine a balloon, with (let's keep it simple) four rays going in from the top, bottom and each opposite side, they would meet in the centre. If each was delivering twenty-five units of stuff, the centre would receive one hundred units, while the space between entry point and centre would only get twenty-five units. Most of the organs in the path of the beam (in Millie's case, the optic nerves) have a tolerance of at least 55 CGE (she is receiving 54 CGE in total, and that's on the tumour bed), but not one single vital organ is receiving more than 52 or 53 CGE, to allow for a margin of error.

Like tiny golden mirrors in the sun, protons from hydrogen atoms will gleam across Millie's vital structures, leaving them almost undamaged, and explode in the most specific and precise manner where their energy is most needed: the tumour bed. Ain't science swell?

## 17) Day 182 – Thursday 3rd October

Millie is doing better every day. She is still a shadow of her former self, physically in particular, but she is improving, so the trend is very much set in the right direction. She is continuing to gain a bit of weight, but more slowly, and we are due to see the endocrine team here in Oklahoma next week to try and grill them on hydrocortisone and its effects (we still think the weight gain is a result of the hydrocortisone she is taking).

At the moment, this most visible effect of her cancer treatment is the one we are finding the most difficult to deal with. We fast-forward the ever-increasing weight in our mind over the next few years, and see an uncontrollable, morbidly obese Millie May scouring for food in every corner of the house. This destiny seems a difficult one to contemplate. We keep reminding ourselves that just because we feel this may be a scenario that will unfold, we won't be able to do much to influence and change the course of Millie's destiny as far as her appearance is concerned. We will just have to focus on good nutrition and plenty of exercise. Talking of which, while waiting for one of her treatments today, I saw her run for the first time since April – playing hide and seek. She ran with another seven-year-old being treated at the centre. There, in the hall. She ran!

*18) Day 183 – Friday 4th October*

I'm feeling low today. I feel low sometimes. It can't be helped and I know it's a feeling that will go away sooner or later. I make it worse by looking back at pictures of Millie when she was well, an innocent seven-year-old girl. I don't care much for justice or fairness during moments like these, but I make a deliberate attempt not to start feeling sorry for Millie or for us. To hell with that! As I recall Millie running, my mind-set shifts, as it has done so many times over the last few months.

It requires some effort, but I am determined not to be a timid friend of truth. I need to accept Millie for who she is and is likely to become, and keep reminding myself that helping her is about fulfilling her potential, whatever that may be, and in curing cancer, ensure she is the best she can be for the rest of her life. I'm up for that. You bet I'm up for that.

# ESTEEM SUCH SCANTINESS
# OF KNOWLEDGE
# OUR DELIGHT

*19) Day 184 – Saturday 5th October*

We have never been seasoned travellers, and had never been anywhere particularly exciting before this trip to Oklahoma City. We would often choose holiday destinations close to airports that had frequent flights back home, and we often cut holidays short. We are at our happiest at home, and I have never understood the need to travel to somewhere else just because it happens to be sunnier than where you live, or nearer to the sea. Other than the health benefits of a boost in iodine and vitamin D, it seems to me to be the most pointless of activities (mostly undertaken, I suspect, to keep up with the Joneses). Travelling is a different activity, though I don't include the absurdities of luxury holidays as a pretence to cultural appropriation. With Oklahoma, we had to admit defeat right from the start. We were going to have to stay for the duration, and this changed the way we looked at our time away. We decided at the beginning that we were going to learn about this place. So much so that the whole family ends up having a fabulous time. During our time we visit places not even

Oklahomans have been to. We've already been to the Science Museum and the zoo, but we also visit the following gems:

- *The National Cowboy & Western Heritage Museum*: America's premier institution of Western history, art and culture. The museum preserves and exhibits an internationally renowned collection of Western art and artefacts to stimulate interest in the enduring legacy of the American West. It also includes a Hollywood room, where I revisit the cowboy heroes of my youth. It takes me back to when I was a boy, some thirty years ago, watching French-dubbed American Westerns with my parents (French TV, for some reason, had a steady release of these Hollywood oldies). John Wayne, Randolph Scott, Joel McCrea, Richard Widmark and James Stewart – there they all are, in a huge 4,000 sq ft room, exploring the various ways the West has been interpreted in literature and film.

- *The Museum of Osteology*: Yup – a museum of bones! Over 7,000 sq ft of bones, skulls and skeletons from all corners of the world, but very educational (as any museum should be) at the same time, so focusing on the form and function of the skeletal system. And not stuffy either. When we buy our tickets, we are told to please *touch the bones*, as they want our experience to be interactive. Imagine that at the National History Museum in London. On the first floor, the museum also shows a movie on a loop about how the carcasses that eventually go on display are cleaned with maggots – my four-year-old boy loves it.

- *Stockyard City*: This is the historic commercial district located in the middle of Oklahoma City. Real cowboys at work every week, the world's largest live cattle auction, authentic Western shops, the West's 'best' steak at

Cattlemen's Steakhouse (where all the presidents go) and craftsmen producing homemade items, from cowboy boots, spurs, hats and clothing to saddles, tack, jewellery and Western art.

- *The Myriad Botanical Gardens:* A jungle in Downtown Oklahoma City, enclosed in a huge glass dome, with its own Millennium bridge going from one end to the other. As it's Halloween time, the gardens come complete with Pumpkinville, and I have never seen so many pumpkins in my life. Millie even ventures on to the small Teletubby-like hills. Anything physical requires effort at the moment, so I rejoice every time I see her do something like that.

They are great museums, but nothing any other big city wouldn't have, especially when you've lived in London for the best part of twenty years. The point about all this is, I suppose, less about the culture and learning, and more that we are doing it as a family, with Millie in tow. And because of the traumatic events of the last six months, we appreciate the simpler things far more. Experiencing this together is what makes it special. Who cares about cowboys? We delight in the *here and now* because Millie's number was almost up – and it may yet still be. But that 'scantiness of knowledge' certainly focuses the mind, and we appreciate the journey all the more, despite the circumstances which bring us here to Oklahoma City.

*20) Day 188 – Wednesday 9th October*

We've been here just over a month now. It's going so quickly. The routine is speeding up time and the weeks are passing at the rate of knots. A usual weekday is normally made up of six units:

- **One**: We wake up at 6am every morning, wash, wake the children up, have breakfast, get ready for school and take all three to Casady, where they have to be in by 8am. With breakfast, Millie has her first lot of medications, including hydrocortisone (2.5mg – 1ml solution of a diluted 10mg tablet in 5ml of water), desmopressin (20mcg – again, this only comes in 100mcg tablets, so we crush, dilute and suction the appropriate amount into another syringe), levothyroxine (50mg – the only sensible drug that comes in a pill of 50mg, so no need to turn the kitchen into a lab for that one) and ranitidine (to counteract the effects of hydrocortisone on the stomach. This is a liquid, and Millie takes 4ml of that). So since Millie has been diagnosed, and given her current daily dose, she has so far taken just under three litres of medicine.

- **Two**: Vanessa takes the children to school and then goes off to do chores (shopping for food normally and making sure that only the purest of organic ingredients enter our bodies...) and then exercise like yoga or Pilates. She managed to find a couple of good studios in the area, and that keeps her mentally balanced, which in turns keeps me sane. Thank you yoga and Pilates. I catch up with work. The time difference means I normally have email correspondence from the UK's morning to deal with, and then I can effectively go through my various to-do lists over three or four hours while the UK is still online. So far, this has worked quite well, and with our third business partner going, there is more and more to be done. I find it frustrating at times not to be there in person, and to leave so much of it on Anna's shoulders, but there is little I can do, and I do what I can to be supportive from 4,000 miles away.

- **Three**: Lunch – my first break. We either go to Whole Foods or have something at home. Vanessa normally goes to pick Millie up from school at 12:40pm. She brings her home and Millie has a break, or they go to the mall, or the supermarket, or the bookshop – whatever. This is the time we give Millie her second lot of medication (desmopressin and hydrocortisone). Millie's energy levels are such that she's been able to do more, and she loves going to bookshops to choose her own books. She seldom reads them, but then who cares. She could if she wanted to and that's what matters. Besides, I remember having a similar fascination with books when I was Millie's age. My mother's philosophy was never to say no to an interest in books, so she would inevitably buy whatever books took my fancy and I would seldom read any of them. Nevertheless, that love for books has remained ever since, and indeed nowadays, reading remains one my favourite activities (non-fiction – I don't care much for fiction, life's too short). I adopt a similar philosophy with Millie and I hope a love of books will endure with her too.

- **Four:** I normally take Millie for her treatment in the afternoon (around 3pm) and Vanessa does the school run. The drive to ProCure takes approximately twelve minutes, with the last half mile along West Memorial Road, a long, straight, undulating road. I can see the centre in the distance, this white sanctuary for the sick, calm and serene on the horizon. It's a peaceful drive and we normally listen to music. For a few minutes I forget the reason why I'm driving or where I'm going, and we both get lost in the ephemeral splendour of moments that will remain forever engraved in my heart. The treatment itself only lasts for thirty minutes and by 4pm we are normally driving back home.

- **Five:** Bath time, teatime and bedtime for the children – in that order. Nothing extraordinary other than giving Millie her third batch of medication, this time very similar to the morning ones (except for levothyroxine, which she only takes once a day). And we give her a much higher dose of desmopressin, spurred on by American endocrinologists who seem to adopt a far more laidback approach to quantity. Millie still gets through at least two nappies a night. It used to be four to six a night, and wet beds every morning in the few months following cancer diagnosis, so there's improvement here (she's now out of nappies). A much higher dose of desmopressin at bedtime seems to improve this significantly, and as her sodiums have been fine over the last six months, we feel comfortable with this approach. If she doesn't drink in the night and she doesn't wee in the night, then her fluid balance must be neutral – at least for the twelve hours she sleeps. No doubt I'll be told off by Millie's endocrinologist, Prof E, back in the UK, but on my head be it – common sense must prevail.

- **Six:** The evenings are spent catching up on the last few work emails, talking to Anna on Skype (she's been staying up until 2am lately to cover for some of the workload), and writing this diary. It seems odd that I write best at night. Most of my best studying (on the rare occasions I did any) was done in the mornings, when my concentration level is at its peak. I have never studied much past three in the afternoon, so I find it a little weird that writing seems to come easier as night falls.

Last week, we asked to see the endocrinologist consultant at the children's hospital. This was for two reasons: the first is that Millie's daily medicines relate entirely to her endocrine dysfunctions and no one has checked her sodium level (I never thought I'd see the day where I actually wanted her sodium levels checked). It seems sensible to make sure we are still doing the right thing with regards to dosage, in particular those relating to desmopressin and hydrocortisone. The second is to get a second opinion on hydrocortisone, to see if the US differed at all from the UK approach (different countries, different protocols) and the consultant's view on possible alternatives or likelihood of her ability to produce ACTH (adrenocorticotropic hormone) being unimpaired.

As soon as we ask for an appointment, ProCure and the children's hospital organise one within half an hour. In addition to this, when the endocrinologist consultant meets us, the first thing he does is give us a business card with his mobile number and email address on it. "Call me any time, email me any time." In contrast, I have to wait two weeks (if I'm lucky, half of the time nothing comes back), for a reply from the endocrinologist at GOSH – lovely, proficient chap though he is. And when we were roaming the wards during Millie's chemotherapy cycles, it usually took a week of chasing to get five minutes of face time. The difference: one is funded by the tax payer through, mostly, tax contributions, the other one is funded by, yup, the taxpayer, but this time mostly through insurance premiums (and partly fiscally, but to a far lesser degree). In the former, the patient is a resident who pays taxes that end up being badly spent, in the latter, the patient becomes a customer – and there lies the distinction. Both are ultimately funded by the same source: us, the ultimate consumer.

Accepting the shortfalls of the US health system, if you can afford it, it is a better service experience altogether. Better service experience doesn't necessarily translate in better equipment, better doctors or a better cure, so let's be careful how we define success here. I am sure with the fullness of time, I will feel less need to contact Prof E as regularly as I want to at the moment, and I understand there are some equally needy children (and parents). But at these initial stages, more responsiveness from the NHS would certainly improve the user interface experience. Most worrying is that this characteristic of the NHS is not a bug, it's a feature, and a recurrent one.

Anyway, back to the consulting room of the children's hospital. The endocrinologist consultant performs the usual tests on Millie, including peripheral vision, and expresses great enthusiasm at the degree of improvement in her functional and peripheral range. He then confirms that if this had happened in the US, she would be on a replacement dose of hydrocortisone, similar to the one she is on at the moment (6mg a day). Like the UK endocrinologist, he doesn't feel hydrocortisone is causing the weight gain, hunger, easy bruising, irregular sleep patterns (need I go on?), but blames surgery and damage to the hypothalamus. Surgery, when I spoke to them, confirmed they did not feel the hypothalamus was damaged and passed the buck to endocrine or chemo. Chemo passed the buck back to endocrine and/or surgery depending on who was in the room (sounds familar?). The endocrinologist feels that changes in eating habits and levels of activity will need to be implemented, as life long lifestyle choices. He also confirms what we have known all along –

that things are still in flux. We are going to need another six to twelve months for Millie's body and functions to stabilise to what we can safely call a base level.

We have noticed that the hunger varies weekly, that some days are better than others, and, dare I say it, that there has been a small cumulative improvement over the last three months. He also tells us she may or may not need hydrocortisone for the rest of her life, but we won't know until we've tested her ability to produce ACTH by herself. Even then, it doesn't mean the adrenals will restart straight away. So back to square one.

There have been so many variables, so many permutations, so many changes, combinations and rearrangements since we started giving Millie her medicines, and so much still depends on the effect of proton beam that we have no choice but to wait it out. My head is spinning. No one can know the mind of God, but something has changed in our outlook. Somehow, this ability to focus on the long-term lifestyle changes and habits for Millie makes her condition more palatable and easier to accept. And as a result of this consultation, we alter the dosage of hydrocortisone to three times a day (instead of four), with two higher doses in the morning and lunchtime, and one smaller one at 5pm. It makes a difference at night. That's something.

# TO THE BEAUTEOUS EYES,
# MINE EYES RETURNED

*22) Day 190 – Friday 11th October*

Millie is halfway through proton beam treatment. She has done fifteen sessions, and has fifteen to go. As I drive back from ProCure, with Millie humming along to 'You Gonna Miss Me When I'm Gone' (otherwise known as 'The Cup' song), my mind goes back to all we have overcome in the last six months, in all of its immensity.

This is just the beginning. The air outside is clean and crisp; the sky, a sea of blue. Clarity and a keen sense of determination invade my thoughts for much of the journey. I will do whatever it takes, for as long as it takes, to get Millie better, and I know Vanessa will too.

*23) Day 194 – Tuesday 15th October*

Every Tuesday, after one of her proton beam sessions, Millie has a follow-up consultation with the nurse/doctor (haven't figured out what she is yet), and the radiologist oncologist consultant. The visit to endocrine confirmed what I had already heard (remember folks, corroboration is validation), that the hypothalamus is not sensitive to radiotherapy of any kind, but *very* sensitive to surgery, so it may well be that some damage was done during the second operation. It is true that some correlation exists between Millie's surge in appetite and that second operation (which is annoying), but at the same time, it doesn't explain all the other associated symptoms she has like sleep irregularity, easy bruising, mood swings – though less so since the hydrocortisone went from 10mg to 6mg and now just 5mg.

I replay back the visit to the radiologist oncologist to test his thoughts. He's not the regular radiologist oncologist and confirms that children with cancers like the one Millie had are normally on hydrocortisone for the rest of their lives. More sitting on the fence ensues. There will be no meeting my saviour today.

I'm bored of talking to the medical profession about ACTH, hydrocortisone, how they never give you a straight-forward answer, or how they often attribute blame to another specialism.


*24) Day 195 – Wednesday 16th October*


Today is a big day for Millie. She is going on her first school trip since the end of that first half term, back in Easter. It seems every week brings something Millie does 'for the first time since it all happened'. I suppose that in itself is a sign of progress. She is going to the Planetarium. Feeling a mixture of concern and excitement, Millie is thrilled at being able to take her own packed lunch, as is Vanessa (she gets to choose what Millie eats – always a source of great satisfaction).

It seems miraculous that she is able to get out of bed, let alone go on a school trip with other children, in the context of the last six months, three brain operations and four heavy cycles of chemotherapy. But there's no miracle here – besides, faith has no substance in my world – just hard grind, orthodox medicine, a brilliant medical team at GOSH and the love of a mother and father who would never give up

She comes back from the trip exhilarated, and my eyes return the gaze of those beautiful eyes.

# AND SUCH ECLIPSE IN
# HEAVEN, METHINKS,
# WAS SEEN

*25) Day 197 – Friday 18th October*

OMG, as my eldest daughter would say, by now in a slight Midwestern twang: only two weeks to go before we return home. It seems that every time we blink, a week goes by.

I decide to write to our UK school's headmaster, Mr M, to confirm we would be back for the beginning of the second half of term. I'm not so worried about Ellie and Luca. They've missed half a term of UK school but have attended the excellent Casady School here in Oklahoma, and have had the opportunity to experience a new culture and make new friends. Millie will require more of a balancing act. To begin with, she has been out of school since 5th April. That in itself is not a concern, but she has undergone the most gruelling treatment over the last six months and has taken a knock both physically and, though it's not necessarily evident at the moment, emotionally.

There are still a lot of moving parts. Whilst Millie's eyesight has come back to full functionality, it is difficult to judge to what degree it has returned, whether it will allow her to sustain the same level of concentration as her peers, if she will require additional support during lessons, or bigger text in exercise books. Proton beam may also have an effect on her cognition, though this is not likely to manifest itself for a few years.

Vanessa and I are keen to reintroduce Millie to normal life, but we also want to protect her against any knocks in confidence she might have in re-joining a class where she will be the smallest (it is now evident she has not grown for a year), but also behind in relative terms to her classmates. If I have to be honest, that is my biggest concern. Lack of knowledge is easily remedied, but a knock in confidence can last a lifetime. I decide not to worry too much about it for the time being, but I air my concern with Mr M, and I have no doubt the school will be supportive and provide the right kind of guidance when it is needed.

The other challenges in reintroducing Millie to full-time school are: a) lunchtime – given her appetite and, it seems, a recently acquired ability to sniff out the fattiest, most sugary food; and b) she still requires medications halfway through the day in the form of pills that need to be crushed and measured. These are important drugs and I need to feel comfortable I can trust the school to administer them in the right way and at the right dose.

Hope, this light of many stars, visits my heart. It is not an emotion I hold dear, but this time I feel it comes more from the effect of merit than of chance. As we look ahead, I hope I continue to have the focus and judgment required to guide Millie over the course of the next few months, as we regain a new kind of normality, and she becomes accustomed to ordinary life once more. That hope I allow myself, because I know it will only be the product of hard grind and diligence from everyone involved.

ProCure closes every year for three consecutive days of maintenance, and those days happen to be next Friday, Saturday and Sunday. So as to keep up with the schedule, they keep the centre open the Sunday before (today). After this session, Millie will have ten sessions left. Five hours of cancer treatment left. It still hasn't sunk in – and I feel slightly apprehensive that we will be leaving. The last two months have been relatively safe: not as gruelling as chemotherapy or craniotomies, so they have allowed Millie to recover. At the same time, we are still *curing* cancer – we are still focusing on an activity that actively reduces malignant cells (or prevents them from growing). After these ten sessions, that's it. We are due to start some form of endocrine support, but cancer treatment will have finished and we will be at the mercy of chance. We can only wait a year and see.

When we leave ProCure, we will be entering a period of shadows, of uncertainty and, ultimately, of worry, at least in the medium term until we find out whether or not recurrence will happen. And yet my vision is clearer than it used to be. I realise as I gaze at the wonderful world in front of me – at Millie, Ellie, Luca and my wife – that I can see better than I did before. In shifting my perspective, this ordeal has enabled me to appreciate what I already have much more, and spend less time agonising over problems I don't have, problems of perception. I just hope I will maintain this outlook in life as we approach each of the MRI scans we have to face in the coming months, and as we establish whether or not Millie's tumour is growing again.

*27) Day 201 – Tuesday 22nd October*

One of my ongoing preoccupations is getting a sense of what Millie May's life (and quality of life) is likely to be in the long term. If she survives cancer, after possible damage and long-term side effects from three brain operations, four cycles of chemotherapy, proton beam irradiation and injury to her pituitary gland and hypothalamus from the tumour itself, how long will she live for? How happy will she be? What will she look like at ten, twenty, thirty years of age? Is she likely to live until she's too old to care? Or will she die prematurely, midway through her life as a result of the condition with which she was afflicted at just seven years of age?

Doctors are reluctant to make predictions about what will happen next week, let alone possible event horizons spanning the next ten years, so I'm getting no luck from them, other than the odd, "I'm still in touch with a few of my previous patients, and some of them have gone to university." Hardly reassuring. The internet is also rather slim and positively negative in this particular area, with most experts quoted in scholarly articles referring to high rates of *morbidity* for such and such condition (they seem to enjoy using that word – it means ill health, illness, sickness. Why not use those words, they seem kinder to people who have already suffered enough). I get depressed reading what I find. Information dished out by charities deals in generalities too broad to be of any use.

I am unable to shift this deep-seated uncertainty about the longer term. Like an eclipse, this obstacle, this black planet of fear, is darkening an otherwise bright(ish) outlook, and it seems reluctant to continue on its elliptical journey. I know when to let go: I shall seek answers another time.

# THE SHADOWY CONE
# ALMOST TO LEVEL ON OUR
# EARTH DECLINES

*28) Day 203 – Thursday 24th October*

ProCure has organised a pumpkin carving activity at the centre and Millie is keen to participate (we're getting close to Halloween). This is due to happen late afternoon, just after her proton beam treatment. While I wait for her in the main reception area, I strike up a conversation with another parent, the mother of a thirteen-year-old girl who is also waiting for pumpkin carving to begin. It turns out that her daughter (who looks eight – but is thirteen) has recently been diagnosed with the same type of tumour as Millie. She is on exactly the same drugs, including hydrocortisone! With the same initial symptoms as Millie had! It occurs to me that this is the first parent I've met who has a child with the same affliction, and I make a mental note to seek out support groups once I am back in the UK, to share our story, our worries, our questions and our concerns.

What's particularly interesting for me, talking to this young girl, is her ability to control her thirst. At thirteen, she is able to monitor and control her intake of water based on the dosage of desmopressin she requires. Millie, on the other hand, aged seven, is unable to control her thirst. I am encouraged by this demonstrable proof of consciousness that develops with age.

This thirteen-year-old girl gives me hope. She is like the north wind, blowing from its milder cheek a blast that clears some darkness from the sky above, and I find the prospect of carving pumpkins significantly less bothersome.


*29) Day 205 – Saturday 26th October*

After fifty-four days in Oklahoma City, the monotony and tedium of our daily routine finally gets the better of my mood. I feel flat today. Lethargy takes hold and I don't feel like doing much. I wait for Vanessa to return with Millie to go for lunch at Whole Foods and sit outside to soak up the last few rays of an Indian summer that is coming to an end.

As I listen to 'If I Go, I'm Goin'', I clear my mind and lose myself beyond time's limits – to happier times, when long was hope, and short was the remembrance of things past and images remote. I know this moment cannot last, but I savour each and every second as I suspend reality, and with it Millie's cancer, for an instant in time and space.


*30) Day 207 – Monday 28th October*

Five sessions (and therefore five days) of proton beam to go! Millie has made progress over the last two months in Oklahoma City, no doubt, but further improvements will be necessary to reintegrate her into normal life. That she can see is a clear bonus – she can go back to the same school as before, but much uncertainty remains, not least as to whether or not cancer will come back.

They almost feel unreal, these twilight hours of cancer treatment, projecting a long shadowy cone towards the flat horizon, and concealing what life might be like when we finally get back home to some semblance of normality.

# THE LOVE THAT MOVES THE SUN AND ALL THE STARS

*31) Day 211 – Friday 1st November*

Today is Millie's last session of proton radiation therapy, and it marks the end of cancer treatment. It is a significant milestone to have reached, and comes after seven months of hard grind for us, and much suffering for Millie. But it's done. Once again, as I have felt many times before, pride overcomes me as I look on at Millie's achievement, at her courage, at her capacity for calm that has given me much comfort and guidance since April.

Next to the reception desk at ProCure there is a brass bell attached to the wall, at eye level. It was a previous patient's gift to the centre, or an 'alumni' as past patients here are called. Next to it, inscribed on a brass plate, is a brief poem:

*Ring this bell*
*Three times well*
*Its toll to clearly say*

*My treatment's done*
*This course is run*
*And I am on my way*

It is a tradition of the centre that when patients come out of their last session, they ring the bell for all to hear. It has chimed often while I have waited for Millie over the last six weeks. And now it's Millie's turn. She will ring it in the next few minutes – as an alumni of ProCure.

A couple of days ago, Millie had her graduation; a ceremony she should have had next week. As we leave for the UK tomorrow they held Millie's ceremony on the Wednesday preceding her end of treatment. Graduation is a big deal here. Approximately four people graduate every week, to become alumni of ProCure, this peculiarly exclusive club. It partly celebrates the achievement of those who have had to walk the long, arduous, lonely path of cancer treatment. Oddly, it's also a marketing opportunity for the centre to 'spread the word', so to speak, about ProCure and its level of customer care. Millie receives a Princess Sofia rucksack signed by all the members of the team, the bead for end of treatment (for her Beads of Courage necklace) and a gold coin with her patient number engraved on it: 1,240.

Millie is too young to recall her story in front of some thirty grown-ups at the graduation, so I do it on her behalf. I have recounted it so many times before that saying it one last time out loud comes naturally: the fuzziness, the blindness, the first diagnosis, the first brain operation, the confirmation of malignancy, the first two cycles of chemotherapy, the acute kidney failure, the hair loss, the second brain operation, the last two cycles of chemotherapy, the third brain operation and two months with my family 4,000 miles away from home for Millie to receive proton beam radiation.

Millie looks on somewhat bewildered, unaware of the magnitude of what she has achieved. I hope this diary will help her, later in life, to understand the enormity of what she has had to endure, and the courage with which she has done it. I know she'll be able read it now, there's just one obstacle to overcome to ensure she reads it free from cancer.

Millie comes out of the double doors that lead from the treatment room into the reception area for the last time. The ones she has passed through some thirty times before. I lift her up so she can ring the bell. And as I gaze at my daughter, ardour and exceeding fondness I have never felt before infuses every cell of my body. Her treatment's done. This course is run and we are on our way.


*32) Day 212 – Saturday 2nd November*


We wake up early to go to the airport. We have spent the last week packing and we are ready to go home. We shut Mary's house front door for the last time. It's still dark outside. We are going to drive to the airport, and one of the lead nurses will meet us there to pick up our hire car and return it on our behalf. The customer first, right to the end.

While we are sad to leave Oklahoma City behind, we are looking forward to going back home. OKC had become a home away from home, but in many ways much more than that. Proton beam is the last phase of what the medical profession calls 'multimodality of treatment' when curing cancer. Our time in Oklahoma has allowed us to regroup after the violence of the first two phases of treatment (surgery and chemotherapy) and is an apt reminder, as we strive to free Millie from this unspeakable disease and the hardship that comes with it, that ultimately, grace can never be found, but must always be earned. I know Millie has been up to the task. I hope I have too.

## 33) *Epilogue to Heaven*

Cancer treatment started in London on 5th April 2013. It finishes here, in Oklahoma City, on 2nd November of the same year. When all is said and done, Millie is clinically in complete remission. That's not to say she's cancer free. We'll have to wait a couple of years before we are certain of that, but she is in a good group overall in terms of chances of non-recurrence. From waking up blind from her first operation, she has regained much of her vision, which was never a certainty, far from it, and she is looking forward to returning to some kind of normality back at home.

If cancer does not recur, the main challenges remaining are those relating to the functions of the hypothalamus and pituitary gland that have been impaired by cancer and its cure. It will take a few months before we establish what level of support she will require in these subtle areas of development. And these are likely to be ever changing. She will certainly be on more than one daily drug for the rest of her life to make up for the deficiencies caused by the illness and its devastating treatment. An illness and related treatment I knew little about up until seven months ago.

I have learned so much since April of this year. I have learnt much about people. I have been blown away by the kindness and compassion that has come our way, from so many and in so many different forms. I hope I will be able to repay in some way the support we have received, from family and strangers alike, who pull together instinctively when cancer strikes a seven-year-old girl, and ask for nothing in return.

I have learnt to accept help without guilt, or the need for immediate reciprocity. I know the time will come when I will have to help someone in return – and I feel reassured that when it does, I will be prepared to assist in a more material way than I would have been able before all this started.

I have learnt to be grateful and humble about our current situation and the support we have received medically and from all those around us. In the last few months, having spent much of my time in places so unrepresentative of normal life, I have met families whose children are going through the most severe of treatments. Treatments that make what we (or rather Millie) have gone through look like a stroll in the park on a warm summer's day.

I have learnt about perspective, and the sense of proportion that invades you when events so overwhelming and traumatic unexpectedly arrive to disrupt the peace and stillness of everyday life.

I have learned that maths and English and the curriculum are really not important.

I have learnt about the need to be functional in our approach to dealing with this devastating illness; it has often required effort on a gigantic scale to see past Millie and her suffering in her darkest moments, and try and focus instead on the long-term tasks ahead.

I have learned to keep optimism in check, and maintain a sense of context about any elements of positive progress we were making. Right from the start, we lived our life one week at a time (sometimes even one hour at a time), and forced ourselves never to speculate, but deal with the facts as and when they arose.

I have learned to trust a remarkable multidisciplinary team at GOSH, who had the best interests of my child first and always. Not that we had any choice, but learning to trust has certainly made life easier. That's not to say you can never challenge the establishment. You should. And I did, whenever mid-level bureaucracy crept in to pollute the professional instinct of people who clearly care about their job and about the wellbeing of others.

I have learned much about Millie, who has suffered on a colossal scale over the last seven months. It will take time to redress that which cancer and its cure has destroyed and damaged. We hope we will be granted a chance at her rebirth. We hope that cancer will not come back. If it does, then difficult decisions will have to be made, and Millie might have to undergo treatment so corrosive that the last seven months will no doubt seem like child's play in comparison. For now, we focus on endocrine, and on rebuilding Millie May small steps at a time. No doubt life would have been a lot harder had it not been for the way in which she has been able to handle it all with fortitude, patience, endurance and an ability to cope with the most gruelling of therapies. She has been *extraordinary* in that sense, and she doesn't even realise it.

And, finally, I have learnt much about myself. After forty-one years of restlessness, having journeyed half of my life's way, it has taken Millie's illness, her wisdom and her guidance, for me to finally be at peace with myself and my surroundings, and gain a new understanding of the world. It turns out that the love that moves the sun and all the stars is none other than that which I have for my children: Ellie Rose, Luca Jack and, of course, Millie May. I know my place now. It's right here with them.

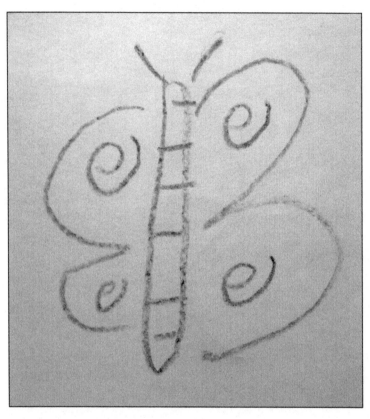

Millie's first drawing since losing her vision, following cancer diagnosis and first brain operation.

A year on, unprompted, Millie puts pen to paper and writes her own version of *Dear Millie*.

When I woke up one moring
my eye's where fuzzy so
my mummy and daddy took
me to the hospetal. I felt a
bit scared. And then we found
out I had a brain tumour
I had to stay
in hospetal a
while to have strong
medason which made my hair fall
off I felt a bit lonley.
I also I had lost of needles

befor tretmant. I had Some lines put in

me, we named them wiggels! because

they where wiggled! all my medesons

whet through my wiggles I also

had to have three operations

(I Loved all the narses)

I went to America to have

my Last tretmant. I went to school
called casady. I made lots of freinds

every afternoon I went to a hospetal

to lie on a bed for 30 minces

very still. after I got a beads

called the "beads of courage" I got

toys too!

and now I have

to have lots of chekups

me feeling beter

but i'm feeling beter!

by millie may x